The
Things
We
Don't
Say

An Anthology of Chronic Illness Truths

May the words in
this book help you
feel much less
alone!

♡ Wendy
Bonner

Julie Morgenlender, Editor

The Things We Don't Say: An Anthology of Chronic Illness Truths edited by Julie Morgenlender.

chronicillnesstruths.com

First edition March 2020.

Published by threebarrelbluff.com.

Published in Las Vegas, Nevada, United States of America.

ISBN: 978-0-578-65432-4 (PRINT)
ISBN: 978-0-578-66400-2 (EBOOK)
Library of Congress Control Number: 2020903712

Chronic illness | disability

Some names and identifying details have been changed to protect the privacy of individuals. The opinions included are those of each author, not of the copyright holder nor publisher. No part of this book should be interpreted as medical or logistical advice.

Cover design by Bob Thibeault: bobtibo7.myportfolio.com/work.
Interior template by bookdesigntemplates.com.
Layout by Kate Estrop: kateestrop.com.

All photos appear by permission of their subjects.

Contents

To my parents, Barbara and David, who have always given me their unconditional love and support. You have gifted me more than I can ever say.

&

To Alie, Hanna, Marisha, and Mimi who have been there through the good times and the bad, always able to make me laugh and there to hold me when I cry.

Introduction

"DOES THIS COUNT AS a chronic illness?" When I asked people to contribute personal essays for this anthology, I was shocked the first time someone asked me this. By the fifth time, I was no longer shocked but still saddened. The fact that so many of us doubt the legitimacy of our health situations due to our stigmatization and erasure by society is exactly why this book is necessary.

I don't remember when I first thought of creating an anthology about life with chronic illness, because in some sense, I have always wanted to do it. Every time I thought about it, it felt necessary and right.

When I first developed symptoms as a child, and for many years thereafter, I looked for community. I couldn't find any. For eleven years I didn't have a diagnosis, so I didn't fit into any of the existing support groups. There was no obvious nonprofit to call. In the early years, there were no blogs or websites to check, no social media to reach out on. When the web eventually became a source for information, I still couldn't find anything helpful for my situation.

These days, there are more places to turn to if you are undiagnosed, but it's still hard to find a place where you fit. And what happens when you have a diagnosis? You still feel isolated. You have doubts. It's lonely. At least, that's how it was for me.

I started an anonymous blog about my own chronic illness feelings and experiences. It has been a great outlet for me to vent my frustrations and joys. It has also provided others with useful information and a sense that they aren't alone in their struggles. I have had many people comment to tell me that they feel the same way about something I described, to say they are glad to know they aren't the only ones, or to simply thank me for talking about the aspects of chronic illness that are rarely, if ever, discussed. I would like to think many more who have never commented are also helped.

At some point I began to think about writing a book about my own situation. I felt there could be value for others in that. But the more I thought about it, the more I first wanted to share other people's voices in addition to my own. I thought about those feelings of isolation and confusion that so many of us have.

I felt that way once before, when I first realized I was bisexual. Then, a couple years after I figured it out, I came across an anthology about being bisexual. The stories felt familiar. I remember thinking, "I'm not the only one!" and it was incredibly comforting. I wanted to provide that feeling of comfort and validation to people with chronic illnesses, too.

As this idea took shape, I realized that not only could people with chronic illnesses benefit directly, but we could also benefit by sharing our journeys with our loved ones. I imagine parents, children, partners, siblings, friends, teachers, and others reading these stories. I imagine someone who has struggled to explain their experiences and feelings to their loved ones handing over a copy of this book and saying, "Please read this particular story. It explains what I have been trying to tell you."

This book contains the truths of our lived experiences, including the ones we rarely share. In the process of creating this book, I asked followers to vote on many potential titles. Each time, there was one clear, outstanding winner: *The Things We Don't Say: An Anthology of Chronic Illness Truths*. This title speaks to people because we want others to understand what we don't say, what we attempt to say, and what we are finally saying in these pages.

I want everyone to find themselves represented here. These personal essays speak about many different topics, many different illnesses, and many different lifestyles. The authors included in this book span different ages, gender identities, sexual orientations, religions, races, ethnicities, and countries of origin. They are parents, siblings, children, grandparents, friends, students, employers, employees, and more. Some write under their real names while others use pseudonyms. My hope is that every reader with chronic illnesses can find at least one author or personal essay with which they identify. That is why every essay includes a short biography, a location, and a headshot of the author. I want you to feel that you know the author and can relate to their situation.

Several people have told me they will share this book with their doctors and medical practitioners. Others want this to be read by medical students. As far as I'm concerned, the more the better! There is so much that society at large does not understand about our daily lives with chronic illness, and I see this book as one small step toward correcting this problem. Please share it with everyone in your life.

I understand that many of us in the chronic illness community struggle financially and therefore cannot afford to purchase a book. Please check your local library for a copy and if they don't have one, request that they buy a copy so that you can borrow it for free. Maybe a friend has a copy that you can borrow. Visit chronicillnesstruths.com/lowcostbooks for more options.

Having authors from around the world means having different forms of English in the essays. While the spelling has all been standardized to American English, you may notice a few British English and Australian English phrases. It is important to me to keep each author's voice intact, so these have remained.

Another intentional choice I made was to not include a glossary of chronic illness definitions within this book. This was beyond my ability at the time of publication. Instead, I chose to make these available at chronicillnesstruths.com/glossary with links to relevant resources. Diagnoses have been defined within each essay where they are necessary to understand the content, but definitions are not necessary for most essays. This approach also has the benefit of being a resource that can be updated over time.

If you would like to know more about me, my diagnoses, or my journey, please read my essays, "This Is Hard" on page 35 and "My Journey for Answers: Because No One Will Care More about My Health Than Me" on page 219, as well as the "About the Editor" on page 239.

Before you begin reading, please keep in mind that the personal essays in this book cover a range of topics and emotions. While you may find some stories uplifting, others may be more difficult to read. Topics include infertility, suicide (particularly in "Pudendal Neuralgia" by Atara Schimmel on page 101), and depression, among others that may be triggering for you. When I first read these stories, I had to pace myself, and I rarely read more than a few at a time. You may need to pace yourself as well. Skip between essays if it feels right. Put the book down and take a break when you need to, as I did. Please be aware that there are several essays that mention sex, particularly "Yes, We Can: Sex and Chronic Illness" by Kit Stubbs, PhD on page 16 and "A Flash of Blue" by Shelia Bolt Rudesill on page 7. There is also profanity in this book. Finally, please remember that nothing contained in this book is medical advice. It is the opinion and experience of the author, and everyone's experience will vary. Please seek professional help as needed.

For resources, additional author information, updates about the audiobook version of this book, merchandise, and more, visit chronicillnesstruths.com. For the bonus material mentioned at the end of this book, visit chronicillnesstruths.com/bonus.

~Julie Morgenlender

Part 1

Relationships: Family, Friends, Dating, & Sex

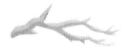

A Flash of Blue

SHELIA BOLT RUDESILL

Pittsboro, North Carolina, United States

MY HUSBAND AND I joyously and thoughtfully wrote our wedding vows. We weren't kids—we were forty-four and didn't want to make promises we couldn't keep. Our love lives had been tough in many ways, and we believed our life together would be wonderland. We leaned together and shared a smile when the pastor said, "There is nothing love cannot endure." We'd waited too long for our soul mates. We vowed that our destinies would be "Woven of one design and our perils and joys would not be known apart."

After three years of marriage our sexual appetites were still insatiable. It was my first marriage and I was delighted knowing that my sexual desires would be met in our marriage bed, or on the dining room table, or under a waterfall in Hanging Rock State Park.

My husband's ex had asked him to leave after a rocky and emotional twenty-three years. When we met, he could tell I was his age and imagined that my life had been as harried as his. He'd been looking for a younger woman without baggage. He said he'd never marry again. But he couldn't resist being loved. When he proposed, he'd hoped for at least ten more years of glorious sex. He got three and a half.

A pain crept into that private part of my body where my legs join my trunk. Intercourse became bloody and unbelievably painful. Soon I couldn't sit comfortably or wear panties or sanitary pads. Tampons were out of the question. I had to switch from toilet tissue to a portable bidet. After visiting several doctors to no avail, I returned to my primary gynecologist with my husband in tow for backup. Previous physicians held little regard that my symptoms were not simply imaginary.

I wanted to scream in anger, but I calmly and emphatically stated, "There is something wrong with me and I'm not leaving the office until you figure out what it is."

The doctor listened to my symptoms again then sat back to think. My shaking hand in my husband's moist palm reminded me of my first dance with a boy at my sixth-grade prom. We'd been nervous, that boy and I, but not to the degree my husband and I were now.

At last the doctor looked up. "I think I know what it is. Will you consent to a biopsy?"

Several days later I crept back to the office alone, hoping for good news. Instead, the stern doctor diagnosed me with lichen sclerosus—small pearly white painful spots on thinning skin of the vulva. As he left the examination room, he paused and looked me in the eye. "You'll never have intercourse again," he said before he closed the door behind him. He left me to cry alone. He didn't have the sensibility or empathy to comfort me. He didn't even send in a nurse to make sure I hadn't flooded the floor with tears or smashed all the medical supplies on the counter. "Ten years of good sex," I heard my husband's jubilant voice say a million times over.

I wept in that stark, cold room. I wept in my hot car. I wept all the way home. I wanted to escape. I didn't want to share my devastating news. I wanted to go back to sixth grade, back to the prom, more self-assured and able to attract the popular boys, marry my high school sweetheart. Then this news wouldn't be so horrible. We'd have had thirty years of healthy, loving sex and this news wouldn't shatter our dreams like a crystal flute crashing onto a marble floor.

I trembled when I told my husband. He smoothed wet curls away from my face and his. The failure of my body made me feel that I didn't deserve him. I didn't deserve to be loved. But he held me in his arms and rocked me like a baby.

I suffered hormonal creams and ointments that only made the diseased tissue worse. I went for a second opinion and then a third. Nothing new. No cure. Only pain for the rest of my life. We took matters into our own hands. These were the days before home computers and Google, so we visited the University of North Carolina's medical library in Chapel Hill where we stumbled onto a little bit of hope. Lichen sclerosus is a skin disease. I called my dermatologist.

He spoke gently—the most caring tone I'd heard from a doctor since this suffering began. I saw hope glimmering. He told me I'd been on the wrong treatment. The estrogen cream prescribed by the gynecologist had only made the condition worse. He prescribed a custom formulated testosterone cream that immediately lessened the pain.

A few weeks later, I met my husband at the front door in the buff. Candles lit the living and dining rooms. I let him lick truffle mousse pâté from my breasts and before we got to the lobster en croute, he was inside of me and we rolled on a sheepskin rug in front of a roaring fire that couldn't come close to matching our cravings. It didn't take more than a couple thrusts before I knew the testosterone wasn't going to cure me. I didn't tell him at first. I pretended to enjoy our lovemaking. I tried to endure until he climaxed. For his sake. Because I loved him so very much.

But I had to cry out and back away when the pain rose to the level of a knife hollowing out my insides like an angler guts a fish.

My husband understood. He was repulsed that he'd inflicted pain on one he loved so much—but it wasn't his fault. There shouldn't have been any guilt but we both felt it. We couldn't give each other what we'd promised.

I wondered how long he'd stay. Wondered and worried. I thought about a friend who, after a hysterectomy, came home to find all her belongings spread across her front yard. Her husband hadn't wanted a "deformed" wife. Another friend suffered breast cancer and finally a mastectomy. Her husband had at least tried to stick around but after a year filed for divorce. He hadn't even looked at or touched her chest since her surgery.

My husband and I went back to the library to search again hoping that, this time, we'd discover a new treatment in one of the more recent medical journals. There was one new treatment: surgery. I called another, younger gynecologist, hoping he would be open for this highly controversial intervention. He smiled when he said, "Let's cut the bastard out! Eliminate the culprit!"

My dermatologist didn't agree. He thought the diseased tissue would grow back. "Besides," he said, "you'll be disfigured."

The ghosts of my friends' ex-husbands haunted me.

I didn't want to leave one stone unturned and neither did my husband, so we opted for the surgery. The young gynecologist teamed up with a plastic surgeon and after two hours and fifty stitches, the lichen sclerosus had been obliterated. My husband and I celebrated with champagne and waited, hoping the revised hardware would work. Six weeks passed. I could now sit comfortably and even wear the kind of sexy and kinky panties that twenty-year-olds receive as gifts at bridal showers. When it seemed right, we tried to show our love for one another in the most intimate and physical way possible. It didn't work. My vaginal opening was about the size of a dime.

We used lubricant and fingers to stretch the tissue. The gynecologist insisted it would stretch so we kept on trying. One day while my husband was at work, I visited a sex paraphernalia shop where I searched for a sex toy that might help with the stretching. I ended up purchasing an item that was the size of a dime at the tip but gradually enlarged to more than the size I needed to be. My husband laughed at my determination and naiveté. I'd bought a butt plug! We got a much needed good laugh out of that, but it turned out to be the perfect instrument. It took a couple months of daily use before we thought my skin had been stretched far enough. We then had painless intercourse for the first time in almost six years. Things were so tight that we joked about having to be physically separated in the ER.

The sex was great for a few weeks until I felt a sharp thorn-like pain protruding through the suture line. Intercourse once again became impossible. In addition to the pain, I found myself in the full throes of menopause with vaginal dryness that even the best lubricant couldn't fix. The sharp pain turned out to be an abscessed Bartholin's cyst, so it was back to the operating room and several more weeks of abstinence.

My body never fully recovered. My husband still looked like a kid in his twenties and had the same sexual desires. He and I tried everything to have normal sex—or maybe I should say spontaneous sex—but it seldom worked. I began experiencing urinary tract infections after intercourse so each event had to be planned and scheduled: a prophylactic antibiotic, a ton of water to ensure I could pee post coitus, lubrication, then finally attempting to be passionate knowing full well that the pain might be too much or that I'd awaken the next day with a urinary tract infection, two more antibiotic pills afterward, and then sitting on the toilet desperately trying to urinate before my husband fell asleep. I wanted and needed to both feel and return his loving touch. More often than not I returned to bed too late, with an empty bladder and an aching heart.

Another year passed. By then, my husband had mild erectile dysfunction, and the knowledge that intercourse was still painful for me worsened his condition. Sex like this is anything but romantic so one day we just quit. The ten years were up anyway. We still held hands and sneaked kisses in restaurants and the movies and grimaced when friends complimented us for still swinging from the chandeliers at our age. We were too embarrassed to tell the truth.

Through all this, I realized how deeply my husband loved me. I remembered our wedding vows, "There is nothing love cannot endure." To him, I was more than my sexuality. He had loved me every single minute. Somewhere in the middle of all this misery and disappointment, my artist husband created the most glorious painting of me with a smile on my face and a twinkle in my blue eyes that flashed beyond the canvas. He could have left me a hundred times. But he didn't leave. He loved me and captured that love on a canvas with the swish of a brush and a flash of blue paint.

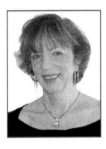 *Shelia Bolt Rudesill is an accidental writer. For forty-five years of pediatric nursing, she dedicated her personal life to the well-being of children. Her writing began at age fifty when she was encouraged to write about her experiences and about those burdened with unreasonable hardships. Since then she has authored five novels and several short stories.*

To the Friend Who Told Me that I Talk About My Illnesses Too Much

R.S. NASH

Melbourne, Victoria, Australia

IT WAS A BALMY night when I was messaging with a friend, and he implied that I talk about my health too much. Imagine my surprise when he then went on to compare his sprained ankle to my multiple chronic illnesses with no cure. I do not blame him for his naiveté, but at the same time it made me rather annoyed.

He wrote, "Do what I do, I wasn't able to walk for two months and I hardly ever brought it up. Focusing on the happy things assists one in seeing the light at the end of the tunnel. Always hold on to your normality. It's the only thing that keeps you sane. Obviously it can be mentioned occasionally; that's healthy."

A tear leaked from my eye as I felt a wave of self-consciousness wash over me. Did I talk about it too much? Is this what everyone thought? Was I driving people away? All these thoughts surged through my mind. But then I came back to the fact that he was basing these statements on inexperience, and I could see where he was getting his point of view from. A lack of firsthand knowledge. I replied saying, "But with all due respect, that's different. I agree to an extent and I see your point of view."

I thought this would end the conversation, agreeing to disagree. But he responded saying that yes it was different to an extent, but the principle was the same. Then he typed a sentence that made me see just how unfounded his argument was. "I do get it though, don't worry," he texted. I laughed at the irony of that statement; if he did understand it then this whole conversation wouldn't have occurred.

After a moment of composure, I wrote back, "Normality does not exist in my life anymore except for my humor and my personality. I cannot walk far. I cannot wash my own hair. On the worst of days I cannot feed myself or brush my own teeth. I have had to alter my life just so that I can have a life. I have lost all independence. With all due respect, it is slightly different to when you are on crutches, and I say this speaking from experience. I am not saying crutches don't suck, but I am saying this is different."

His only response to that was the audacity to dare me not to talk about my illness for a day, to which I retorted, "Does this include when I need someone to wheel me to the toilet? Or when I desperately need a drink but can't get up? Or when people ask what's wrong with me?" The conversation faded after this response, and we have never talked about that conversation since.

Dear friend, I am not angry at you for your ignorance. It is not your fault that you do not understand that my illness is every moment of every day. That I have to calculate whether I have enough energy to make it to the toilet and back. That I have to carry my phone with me on that short journey to the toilet in case I collapse. That every single move I make has to be calculated. It is not your fault that you would not see how there is no "light at the end of the tunnel" for me like there is for you. That my normality has had to be redefined in a way you could never imagine. Do you still not see? This is why I will continue to talk honestly about my illness. Because misconceptions and conversations like ours still happen to other people like me. To my friend who told me I talk about my illnesses too much, I will continue to do just that, and I hope you can one day see why.

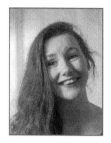

R.S. Nash is a twenty-year-old from Australia living with multiple chronic conditions. She likes to advocate and raise awareness through art and writing, and is passionate about helping reduce stigmas surrounding chronic illnesses.

Yes, We Can: Sex and Chronic Illness

KIT STUBBS, PHD

Somerville, Massachusetts, United States

HI, I'M KIT! My chronic illnesses are generalized anxiety disorder and fibromyalgia syndrome, which I've been living with for more than ten years. One of the pain management techniques I learned early on was distraction; if I could give my brain enough other sensations, the pain signals couldn't get through. Having sexy times with my partner provides a lot of fun feelings to focus on. If I can reach an orgasm, it's super effective.

I recognize that sex isn't an option for everyone. Some asexual folks don't enjoy sex, which is fine! And for sexual folks, the physical and/or emotional barriers one must overcome to engage sexually with themselves or partners may be too high. If you're interested in trying though, here are three things I've learned about having an enjoyable sex life, despite my challenges:

1. My partner and I give ourselves permission to redefine what "counts" as sex. In the United States, most people think of sex as "penis-in-vagina (PIV) intercourse," and other sexual activities are sidelined as "foreplay." This definition is problematic not only because it excludes queer people, but also because it puts all the emphasis on one particular activity—

an activity that my body might not be up for on any given day. Instead, I think of sex closer to how artist Erika Moen defines it, "Being intimate in an arousing or stimulating way with someone else."[1] Suddenly, the doors are thrown open. There are all kinds of activities that my partner and I can give and receive pleasure by doing, and I don't have to stress out over whether I can do that One Particular Thing. Plus, if we're engaged in arousing activity X and my body decides that it's had enough of X, we can just try switching to something else. No big deal!

2. I play to my strengths. Since I'm not stressing out over whether my body can do One Particular Thing during sexy times, I can consider a wide range of activities to see what might work given how I'm feeling. If genital penetration feels like too much energy or effort, maybe I'll try some oral sex instead. If I think I'd like to try for an orgasm, I use a vibrator to help me since it's too physically stressful on my hands and arms not to use one (and I don't let myself feel bad about that). If I'm feeling low-energy, I'll invite my partner to watch some sex-positive porn together—Tristan Taormino's *Chemistry* series is my favorite. Maybe we'll each touch ourselves while watching, maybe I'll help my partner get off, or maybe I'll find I have more energy than I had thought, and we'll try something more involved.

I'm also interested in BDSM (bondage, domination, sadism, and masochism) and like to play with power dynamics. I know some folks with fibromyalgia find that receiving pain through BDSM play is very helpful; for me, I live with enough pain that adding more, even in an erotic context, just isn't fun. If my partner wants to receive

---

1 From the comic "What is Sex?" in *Oh Joy Sex Toy* by Erika Moen and Matthew Nolan.

intense sensations, I can't use popular toys like paddles or floggers because they're too physically demanding. Instead, I look for sensation toys that don't require upper body strength. I've found I can get a lot of mileage out of clothespins, clips and clamps, micro bondage with yarn, and bamboo skewers. No toys within reach? Biting (consensually, of course) has also worked well for me.

The key to making this work is communication with my partner. I make sure to let them know where I'm at, physically and emotionally, and I try to suggest activities that will be fun without being too challenging for me. If we're doing something and I need to stop or change positions, it's okay to say so. We've agreed that it's more important that both of us are enjoying what's happening than for us to keep going while uncomfortable for the sake of the mood. Plus, I'm more turned on when I'm able to relax, and that makes my partner more turned on, too.

3.   I try to stay open to being turned on, even if I don't feel like I have much of a sex drive. While I think about sex frequently as part of my work, it's rare for me to be overcome with the feeling that I want to have sex right now. There are lots of reasons why someone might not become hungry for sex the way they become hungry for food (such as medication side effects, stress, or pain levels, to name a few.) Rather than worry about why I'm not feeling hungry for sex, I've found it's better to keep myself open to the possibility of sex.

If something happens that might lead to sexy times— whether it's my partner's suggestion, or I'm reading something erotic, for instance—I first pause to assess where I'm at physically and emotionally. Sometimes the idea of sex is completely unappealing, and it's completely okay if I don't want to pursue it. Much of the rest of the time, even if I'm not turned on right at that moment, I encourage myself to relax, try some sexy activities, and just see what happens.

"Let's go upstairs, make out a little, and see what happens," is what I will say to my partner. As the ball gets rolling, if I find that I become more relaxed and turned on, then I'll be interested in even more sexy activities. I can't tell you the number of orgasms I've had that I wasn't really expecting, where play started with, "No guarantees, let's just see." At the same time, my partner and I accept that sometimes make outs are just make outs, or maybe only one of us will have an orgasm, and that's also completely okay.

Learning to have an enjoyable sex life while dealing with chronic illness has meant lots of communicating with my partner. Together, we've made a lot more activities part of our sexy times, and I focus on activities that work well with my body's capabilities. I don't stress out over my libido or over the fact that I need to use toys to reach orgasm. Instead, I encourage myself to relax and see what happens.

If you'd like to become more engaged with your sexuality, whether you have a chronic illness or not, I hope you'll consider these perspectives and use what works best for you.

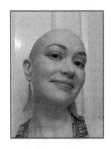

Kit Stubbs, PhD, is a non-binary/queer/femme roboticist, maker, and entrepreneur who is more interested in people than in technology. Kit earned their PhD in robotics from Carnegie Mellon University and later founded the Effing Foundation for Sex-Positivity (effing.org), a 501(c)(3) nonprofit whose mission is to reduce sexual shame by fostering sex-positive art and education. They blog about technological empowerment for sexuality and pleasure, including their experiences and creations, at toymakerproject.com. Kit also co-organizes teasecraft-boston, a meetup group for sex/ kink-positive crafters (teasecraft.com).

Multiple Sclerosis: My Lost Connections

SÓNIA LOPES

Lisbon, Portugal

I WISH SOMEONE WOULD have told me that I was going to lose people when I was diagnosed with multiple sclerosis. Doctors, nurses, therapists, books—I had access to a lot of information and the health care professionals around me were excellent. But no one told me that the social aspect of living with a chronic debilitating disease like this would be the hardest for me to manage.

People have very different coping styles, and everyone reacts differently to the news. My parents, for instance, went into overprotective mode until I eventually told them I would rather not have them calling three times a day to check on me. But overprotective, I was about to find out, would sound really nice once I realized some of the people closest to me were going to be dismissive, insensitive, and disrespectful.

It takes a healthy amount of maturity to deal with such a condition. If you're the patient, you're going to have to do a little growing up whether you like it or not. If you're the friend, colleague, boyfriend, husband, or employer, you may think you can get away with remarks meant to be funny—they're not actually funny. That was my first bad experience with someone. I was worried about some medication I'd started that was messing up my liver, and I was considering cutting out some foods. My friend nonchalantly says, "As long as you don't have to cut out sex you'll be fine." What the . . . ? I was sensitive because this was a month or two right after the diagnosis. Honestly, sex was the furthest thing from my mind. If it was meant to be funny, almost three years later I still don't see what the joke is.

Then comes the cool boyfriend. He had a different way of dealing with my condition, by basically ignoring it. I don't know if he hid his head in the sand because it hurt him to see me struggling, or if he hoped that by dismissing my symptoms and pretending I wasn't ill I would miraculously be cured. That obviously didn't work very well because I'm still ill. He used to tell me that it wasn't easy for him, either. Well, you don't go around telling this to people who are chronically ill without educating yourself about the illness they're living with. You can't expect them to manage an awful lot of things by themselves and also make it easy on you.

The thing is, he never did educate himself. There's the internet, there's books, there's patient groups, etc., and then there he was, blissfully ignorant. He said things to me like, "You're tired already?" He pushed me far beyond my fatigue, and even accused me of faking symptoms because I was spoiled, wanted attention, and wanted to get my way.

Then there's the other friend. The one who, no matter how many times you tell him about your condition, your symptoms, your limitations, still makes you feel like you have to explain yourself. That you have to apologize for being the way you are, for not being able to go out as many times as they'd like, for not being able to soothe his loneliness while you're trying to keep your own head above the water. It's exasperating to go over the same issues repeatedly, only to have the other person disregard them completely. If this isn't a toxic relationship, I don't know what is.

I chose to let go of these people, some of them gradually, some of them more abruptly. And it hurts. As if you don't have enough on your plate already, you also have to anticipate how interactions with people, some of them people you thought would be there for you through thick and thin, are going to be. You plan for how much to disclose when you meet someone new. So much for spontaneity.

Multiple sclerosis happens when your immune system attacks the myelin sheath that insulates your nerve fibers, causing the connections between neurons to be impaired or permanently lost. For me, it has also caused my relationships with people to be temporarily impaired—or permanently lost.

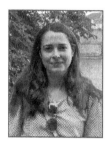 *Sónia Lopes lives in Lisbon, Portugal, and has been working in publishing for over a decade. Among some of her passions are contemporary dance, writing, and traveling, but mostly she's just happy to spend time with close friends and family and enjoy a glass of red wine.*

This I Believe

MARCIA ALLAR

Newton, Massachusetts, United States

I'VE BEEN SICK FOR more years than I have been well: thirty well, thirty-one unwell. I believe what keeps me alive is the island of friendships I have been lucky enough to keep. My friends are like the candy Life Savers I used to eat, and they do save my life time and time again. Like the candy, my friends come in different tastes and colors.

My oldest friend was once my head nurse and my newest friend is a former childhood friend I reconnected with through Facebook. I find that the older my friends are, the better the taste and color of Life Saver they are for me. They are the cherry, pineapple, and mango flavors. Most of these tasty friends knew me when I wasn't sick. They hold the containers of hope for me that I might feel better again someday or somehow. I borrow these containers of hope, courage, strength, faith, and the power of the possibility of better health to ward off my feelings of despair, helplessness, and isolation.

I am an extrovert by nature, and now I'm stuck at home with no place or people to "vert" with. My friends find a day every month or two to come visit me, or they'll make a phone appointment with me to break the never-ending stress of doctor appointments and being on the couch. They say I help them as much as they help me, but there is no comparison. When I feel like I am drowning, a short conversation brings oxygen back to my water-filled lungs. We can talk about our now-grown kids, or other stressors and I can feel normal, as if I too were in the world.

Some have enormous empathic capacity to get what my daily life is like. Others less so, but I imagine the enormity of it all can feel consuming and scary for them. Even though I am not contagious, there is a natural self-protection in us all to need to take a break or stay away from another's pain at different times. Over the years I finally learned that and don't withdraw or feel hurt after their plans change. I have learned that I can't expect impossible certainty or availability of anyone or anything. I now accept that I need to be the initiator of these "play dates" or phone calls, as they are married or have partners and have, thankfully, full and healthy, busy lives.

I make sure my Life Saver candies are stocked up and book my "play dates" in advance so that I don't have to go a whole weekend in total silence. Or a week with no one to talk with or see. I have also noticed that some of my friendships have faded just like the taste of some Life Savers; suddenly it doesn't feel or taste good. But then sometimes, that flavor is good again—much to my surprise, as relationships are always moving and changing. I am grateful and thankful to have my friends in my life to keep me afloat, just like a lifesaver, and help me to keep putting one foot in front of the other in this crazy thing called life. This I believe.

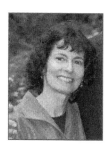

Marcia Allar lives with complex regional pain syndrome, chemical sensitivities, Ehlers-Danlos syndrome, and osteoporosis. She was an oncology head nurse and then a trial attorney for severely injured people in Boston, Massachusetts. She now provides environmental counseling regarding healthy homes, nontoxic products, clean water, and safe foods. She lives in Newton, Massachusetts with her beloved dog, Sophie, and is the mother of two adult children, Sarah and Ben.

One-Two Punch

CHARITY COLE

Royal Oak, Michigan, United States

CHRONIC ILLNESS SEEMS TO have followed me my entire life. I grew up with a mom who lives with depression and fibromyalgia. I survived that only to be diagnosed with multiple sclerosis (MS) in my late teens. Multiple sclerosis is an autoimmune disorder affecting the central nervous center, including the brain and the spine, so just about everything if it wants to. For me, it affected my balance and use of my right hand.

"It was really cool having to use a cane in high school," said no teenager ever.

My college years were also full of MS problems with walking and writing, but I tried not to let it slow me down. I still paid my way through school, had friends, and graduated with honors. I worried no one would ever love me and want to marry me with my baggage though. The fifteen hospital stays during my twenties seemed to bear that out. Why would anybody want to take on living with and loving someone who was in and out of the hospital every month or so?

Then I met someone! He didn't seem scared of all my stuff, rather, he focused on other things like, here was this girl who was sometimes in a wheelchair currently running around the zoo to catch up with a group of friends—yup, running. Through a friend we found a doctor who treated the MS proactively, without hospital stays. I got a little more stable and we planned our wedding. My face was round on our wedding day from the latest course of steroids I had to do, but I walked down the aisle toward my soon-to-be husband that day, and all over Disney World for the next week.

Over the next two years, I continued to do intravenous therapies of steroids to keep the MS at bay. I started to feel better for longer periods of time. I dreamed of a family. The doctor agreed I was stable enough to go off my medications for six months, and then we'd talk again. We found out we were expecting a child two months later and I've been in remission for the ten years since. I have required no treatment or dmedication for the MS since July of 2005. When my doctor said, "Well, maybe you have a mild course of the illness," I laughed. Fifteen hospital stays in two years, two of them a month long, involving learning how to walk again. Mild? When I asked him how this was possible, my doctor said, "We know hormones play a role in starting MS, and sometimes they play a role in stopping it."

I danced with my two oldest girls, packed away my wheelchair, and just had fun as a mama. I was home free, until my third daughter was born. Her birth brought postpartum depression and anxiety, and ultimately more chronic illnesses: bipolar disorder and generalized anxiety. Bipolar disorder is characterized by periods of depression—feelings of despondency or dejection—and mania—great excitement, euphoria, agitation, and over-activity.

Like the MS, bipolar disorder has brought hospital stays. My first was just weeks after my youngest was born. I had started some medication for the depression and anxiety after she was born. It helped a little, so my midwife and I decided to up the dose. That did not help. Suddenly, where I had been antsy, I could no longer stop moving at all. One evening while on the new, higher dose, I cleaned my entire house in five hours, including changing the baby out of her cloth diaper so I could clean all the laundry. It all *had* to be done.

The next day I had one thought, "Get the girls to my midwife, she can take them and love them, and I can just disappear." This thought grew and grew until it pushed all others out. I took my shower, packed up the girls' favorite items, and got us all in the minivan. Off to my midwife we went. "I need to see her. I'll wait, but I have to see her," I pleaded when I got to her office.

I didn't wait long. She hugged me as I sobbed into her shoulder and asked her to take them home and love them. Instead she got my kids playing in another room so they wouldn't get scared, she called my hubby, and got me help. I headed to the hospital via ambulance for the psychotic break I was experiencing.

The horrors of that stay began as soon as I arrived. There was a small dingy room filled with garbage and litter where they did my body search. The peeling paint and gross bed did nothing to brighten the room or my mood. My tears were endless. The nurse kept saying, "If you want to get home, you can't cry in front of the doctor." Not cry? How in the hell was I supposed to do that? I was away from my beautiful baby, away from my family, and didn't understand what was going on.

I saw four psychiatrists in twenty-four hours. The first wanted to up my medication. The second recognized I needed to be taken off that drug. The third told me I didn't have postpartum depression because I didn't fit what his book said and that I couldn't expect him to spend so much time with me. He also yelled at me to stop crying. The fourth said I wasn't a risk to anyone or myself and I should go home. So, home I went, with no treatment plan of any kind or any idea what to do next. I got home feeling more lost and distraught than I had when I went to my midwife. I had used up my one chance at help. Now what?

I did the only thing I knew to do, I called my midwife again. She found me a doctor who specialized in postpartum mood disorders who could see me that day. He was unconventional, his manner was a little off-putting, but only my husband noticed those things. What I saw was a glimmer of hope. He sent me home with a fistful of medication samples and an appointment for two days later. I worked with him for seven months. In that time, we tried a myriad of medications and a couple of alternative therapies. Nothing worked well. By this time, I had noticed his odd behaviors and was more than a little frustrated with him. He had taken me off all my medications after one of his failed alternative therapies and I survived two months like that, then I needed help. Badly. My midwife tried, but we both knew this was beyond her scope of care, so I once again went searching for a psychiatrist.

I was turned down by one clinic because by this time my baby was over a year old, so I no longer qualified for the postpartum program. A coworker found me sobbing after that call and gave me the name of someone she knew. He agreed to see me just a couple of days later.

I spent a year working with him to get my medication right and a good basis of a therapy plan. I had two more hospitalizations, but things were finally improving—then I lost my job and the insurance he accepted. That was three years ago. I am no longer able to work. My youngest is now five years old, and life still isn't quite what I expected it to be after her birth. I take two handfuls of medications a day just to keep me somewhat even, and yet my days are still filled with seesawing emotions that stem from the early days of her life.

I've seen some improvement since being home. Things aren't perfect. The doctors I am now seeing are still desperately trying to get my treatment right, a complex combination of medications and therapy strategies, but now I am able to rest when I need to, I can take the necessary medications that I could not while working due to side effects, and I am surrounded every day by the reasons I fight the mental illness: my three daughters, their beings, their smiles, their laughs, their love.

They help me find the strength to wake up every morning, fight back the dark thoughts of depression and death, or slow down the speed of my thoughts when mania hits. When either struggle comes to the forefront, my thoughts seem to get very loud with either darkness or activity. I have a hard time coming out of those thoughts; I get stuck and obsess over the speed and darkness of my thoughts. Things may be hard in my mind, and then one of my girls will ask for a hug or a kiss and I am here again. I am with them, maybe not for long, but for that moment, I can breathe. If even for just that moment, I am free.

A moment may not seem like much, but when the dark days and the manic days string together in a necklace of unending struggle, those moments become something to live for, they become little bits of light in a mind of darkness and struggle. And I'll take it; I'll take every moment of hope, every bit of distraction, every ounce of my friends' and family's love to get through this thing called chronic illness. I'll take it.

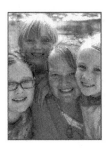

Charity Cole is a stay-at-home, homeschooling mom who shares her story of living with chronic illness in hopes of encouraging other parents that you can live and parent well while facing ongoing health challenges. She blogs about faith, family, homeschooling, and chronic illness at gigglesandgrimaces.com.

Part 2

Experiencing the Emotions

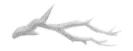

Imagine

MICHAELA SHELLEY

Spartanburg, South Carolina, United States

Imagine...
A life filled with
hospitals,
doctors,
needles,
and pain.

Imagine...
being told you have this disease.
What if that disease had no treatment?
No surgery, no magic pill, no chance of remission,
and there is no cure.

Life would never be the same
That perfect happy life I once had
no longer exists.
It's like my life was sucked into a tornado
then spit back out again
and shattered into a million and one pieces.

Imagine...
what it feels like

to run on nothing.
Your energy level hits rock bottom.
It's like two double A batteries trying to run a car
Doesn't work well... does it?

Imagine...
watching your body fail
your organs dying one by one
but your mind is still alive.

I don't have to imagine.
This life...
Is my reality.

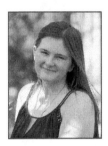

Michaela Shelley is a college student living with mitochondrial disease. She writes about her and her brother's experiences with the disease on her blog: chronicallyawesome23.blogspot.com.

This Is Hard

JULIE MORGENLENDER

Concord, Massachusetts, United States

LIVING WITH CHRONIC ILLNESSES is hard. Very hard. That's the part no one wants us to talk about. Instead, society prefers to see us as inspirational. I hear that all the time. How inspirational that I am smiling and laughing when I'm happy, as if they expect me to be sad and crying all the time. How inspirational it is that I am helping a friend with a problem, as if they expect me to spend my days staring at a wall and not talking to anyone. How inspirational it is that I haven't given up, as if they expect me to have to killed myself when things first got hard.

And you know what? Hearing that is hard. I hate it when people tell me how inspirational I am just for living my life. If they want to compliment me for an actual achievement, like creating this book, that's great. But I am insulted and hurt when people tell me how great I am for continuing to live.

Hearing platitudes is hard. I don't believe this happened for a reason. I don't believe some higher being has a special plan for me. I don't want to hear that a cure or treatment is "right around the corner"—I stopped believing that twenty years ago. I don't want someone else who has never experienced anything like what I live with every day telling me that they believe it's for the best. That doesn't help me; it only hurts.

Not knowing what tomorrow will bring is hard. I make plans with friends, always adding, "If I feel up to it" at the end of the message. Sometimes I do everything "right." I rest up in advance, eat good foods, take extra medications, and still, half an hour before I need to leave—after I have already gotten dressed up and am ready to go—I have to cancel. I have missed ordinary outings with friends, birthday celebrations, going-away parties, a bachelorette party. I have canceled many dates. It's one thing to cancel a date when I'm in a committed relationship, but when I'm just starting to date someone it's much harder. Canceling a first or second date, even when I try to reschedule, is a sure way to end a relationship before it even begins. Once, a good friend invited me to a wedding, and I knew I couldn't handle both the ceremony and the reception, so I asked which one he preferred me to attend. He chose the reception. I went and had a great time for about an hour, but before dessert had been served I just couldn't manage it any more. I went home, exhausted, sick, and upset that I couldn't even manage the wedding reception. How is anyone supposed to have a social life when they never know which days they will feel up to leaving the house, or for how long?

Not knowing how my health will progress (or not) is hard. For a long time I developed pain in a new set of joints every couple of years. Then, recently, I developed pain in three new sets of joints within just a few months' time. I was more upset than I can express. I was in so much pain that it was hard to function. At the same time, I was constantly worried: Was this the beginning of the end for my joints? Would I experience more rapid deterioration now? What would happen when I couldn't use my hands anymore? How soon would I have to give up my favorite activities, some of which had suddenly become extremely painful? Would I ever be able to enjoy sex again, or would that, too, become too painful? The thoughts whirled and there were no answers—only fear.

Having to depend on others is hard. I have always been independent. I am thankful that I can still live on my own, but I question how long that will last. I hate having to ask for help, but there are many things that I simply cannot do. It's not a matter of willpower. Sometimes it's carrying something heavy. Sometimes it's using a hammer on a nail. Always, it's hard to rely on others.

Making difficult medical decisions is hard. Should I take the medication that will cause infertility, the medication that will likely lead to brittle bones and cancer, or the medication that gave me panic attacks the last time I took it? That wasn't a fun choice, and certainly not an easy one, either. I am constantly having to make difficult decisions that only I can make. I can ask for advice from doctors, friends, and family, but in the end, I am the one who must choose a treatment, a test, a doctor. And it's hard, because the wrong choice could have dreadful consequences, and "do over" is not an option.

Being honest is hard. I spent my life pretending that things weren't as bad as they really were. The pain started when I was twelve, lasting for weeks or months before going away, only to one day return again. I learned at that time that if I talked about it too much, grown-ups stopped listening. When I was sixteen the pain changed. It became more severe and also unending. I had pain twenty-four hours a day, and learned quickly that I had to ask for certain accommodations, like note takers in class for when I couldn't hold a pen, but if I asked for too much I would be questioned about ulterior motives. One doctor said I was making it up for attention. Another said I was imagining the pain and sent me to a psychologist. I spent my adult life not letting on how much pain I was in. I talked about it occasionally, but not often. When I said I couldn't do something, people often looked at me like I was making it up, exaggerating, or just being difficult. That still happens, and that's super hard in and of itself.

I learned to put on a smile, even when I was in pain. I recently found myself near tears as I told a friend about all of the new pain I was experiencing, but then I changed the subject. When he talked about his own life, I found myself smiling, even though I was miserable. I tried to stop smiling, but didn't know how. I wasn't happy, but after twenty-seven years of pain, I knew how to pretend the pain wasn't there. When I could no longer work due to my symptoms, I found myself having to not pretend, and didn't know how to stop. The lawyer needed to see how things really were. The insurance investigator who interviewed me was watching for signs that I was faking. The doctor who worked for the insurance company was also watching for signs that I was faking. And worst of all, I felt like I *was* faking because, for the first time in decades, I wasn't pretending. I was doing my best to show how I really felt. And that was one of the hardest things I had done.

Living with the guilt is hard. There's the guilt that I don't help others as much as I want to. The guilt that I no longer work full time. The guilt that I'm too sick to do so many things. The guilt that I'm not as sick as others. The guilt that I have to ask others for financial help. The guilt that I'm in a better financial situation than others. The guilt that I can't take care of myself 100 percent. The guilt that I can take care of myself better than so many others. The guilt that I can't leave the house every day. The guilt that I can leave the house at all when so many others can't. I grew up with Jewish guilt, but chronic illness guilt is so much harder.

Imagining the future is hard. If I am this ill in my thirties, what will my fifties be like? How about my seventies or my nineties? I can't fathom any of it. How much more pain will I be in? How much worse will my fatigue and other symptoms be? Will I be able to take care of myself? I have a strong support system, and I am grateful for that, but what happens when I can't rely on them? Older relatives will pass away. Friends will move away. I am unmarried and don't know if that will ever change. How will I survive in a way that I can still be happy?

And yes, sometimes getting through the day is hard. Sometimes the fatigue, the nausea, the pain are so bad, I can hardly move. Sometimes I wonder if it would be easier to die. Sometimes I can't eat, I can't read, I can't do my favorite hobbies like crochet. Looking at social media is emotionally painful as I see my friends doing all of the things that I can no longer do, and will probably never be able to do again. Watching TV is hard, as I don't have the focus to watch something new or the patience to rewatch something I have seen before. On those bad days, I watch the seconds tick slowly by, waiting until it's time to go to bed. And then I wake up, having to do it all again.

Yes, living with chronic illness is hard. I still find happiness and joy in life, but I wonder sometimes if those who aren't as close to me, who don't hear me talk about the hardest parts, see the happiness and joy and don't realize just how hard it is, too. Because it is. This shit is hard. That's why I need to focus on and appreciate the days that aren't quite as hard. Because those better days are the times that pull me through. Even when they're hard.

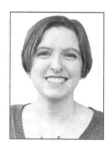

Julie Morgenlender is a friend, daughter, aunt, crocheter, reader, creator of this anthology, and so much more, despite being unable to work full time. She enjoys walking in the sunshine, petting dogs, and spending time with awesome people. She volunteers for her chronic pain support group and is on the board of directors of the Bisexual Resource Center.

I Didn't Cry on My Birthday This Year

TARA A.
Alexandria, Virginia, United States

MY STORY WITH THIS all started in 2008, when I became very sick with a wide variety of symptoms that were eventually diagnosed as chronic fatigue syndrome/myalgic encephalomyelitis (CFS/ME). The fibromyalgia diagnosis came a little later, and since my CFS/ME symptoms are much stronger and much more present than the fibromyalgia pain now, I tend to identify more with CFS/ME. Since 2008, I have seen twenty-four different doctors; had three surgeries; multiple biopsies, X-rays, CT scans, MRIs, EKGs, and ultrasounds; an EEG; an echocardiogram; a colonoscopy; an endoscopy; and more that I'm forgetting. I have tried a variety of different diets, routines, and programs. I have also tried hundreds of different medications, supplements, and vitamins.

I don't talk about the details of my illness all the time and I always try to put on a brave face. This is how I cope with it. But I also know that it's hard for those around me to really understand what I go through when I don't talk about the details and when I look relatively normal. I think that's the hard part for me. When I look sick and can't get out of bed, it's a lot easier for them to understand than when I look completely normal but feel sick. I also have more good days now than before, so I can get out and do a little more, which can be a double-edged sword. I can so easily do too much and pay for that, and when I'm out of the house and look normal, it's even harder for others to understand how sick I am.

This illness has changed my life in so many ways. I would give every penny I have to recover completely. I went from a highly functioning person with a very full and busy life and career to someone who has been housebound for months at a time. I have lost many things, like the job that meant so much to me; the career I worked so hard to build over the course of a decade; the ability to work even on a part-time schedule; the ability to travel often and to places further than a few hours away; the ability to do most physical activities; my ability to spend time outside in the warm months; my independence; my ambition. I have missed so much—weddings, funerals, showers, births, parties, trips, and most of my thirties. I've also lost many relationships, simply due to the fact that I cannot attend a lot of events and I constantly cancel or change plans because I don't feel well.

I have had to drastically limit what I do and who I see. I learned quickly that being around people who don't want to at least try to understand what I'm going through doesn't work for me. I have lost all tolerance for sick-shaming, listening to someone compare my symptoms to how tired they are because they had a busy week or have kids, and people with a lack of empathy. I no longer engage with anyone who tries to debate the reality and severity of any invisible illness, tells me that going gluten free cures everything (it doesn't), or tries to convince me (a life-long vegetarian) that I need to eat meat to recover. It was shocking at first to have to deal with these types of people daily, but I'm used to it at this point and just say good riddance to them.

It has been a very difficult time and something that I never imagined dealing with. I am improving, so very slowly, and what I'm able to do has increased each year. I do have a group of serious supporters, consisting of friends and family that have been on this roller coaster with me, and they are there for the bad times as well as the good. My daily buddy, a sassy miniature dachshund that showed up in my life at exactly the right time, does all that she can to make me smile and want to get out of bed each day, almost like she knows what I need. I know I could not do this alone.

And yet, I often feel so alone. There is a very real ache of loneliness and otherness, a sadness around missing out on so many life events, and a fear of causing a flare or relapse that surrounds me at all times, like a heavy fog that only I can see and feel. I live in a constant state of thinking and measuring and planning, trying to have as much of a life as I can without overdoing it. It can make a person feel crazy. Along the way, I found an online CFS/ME group that provides a regular dose of compassion, empathy, knowledge, and support that has been a lifeline for me. With that group, I feel understood and less alone. But that group exists online, and my personality demands some sort of in-person experience to feel alive and understood.

Enter the MEAction group and the #MillionsMissing campaign of May 2016. MEAction is a group of patients and advocates working together to fight for health equality for CFS/ME by raising awareness and demanding support for a drastic increase in federal funding for CFS/ME research and testing. The #MillionsMissing campaign was launched to represent the millions of people with CFS/ME that are missing from their careers, families, and schools because they are so debilitated; the millions of dollars in federal funding for research and clinical trials that are missing for this disease; and the millions of doctors and practitioners who lack the knowledge and training to provide quality care for CFS/ME patients. This campaign involved a virtual protest, in-person protests at various offices for the Department of Health & Human Services, and meetings with staff from various legislators' offices.

I just happened to click a link on Facebook and decided to volunteer wherever I could, without even knowing exactly what I was signing up for. I had to do it that way; if I had really thought about it, I would have been too anxious and would never have gone through with it. I ended up participating in all aspects of the campaign and was shocked at how it affected me. For starters, after weeks of rain, the weather changed overnight to the extremely hot and humid Washington, D.C., summer that slaps you in the face every year around that time. In addition, I had three days of activities, multiple trips from my home in northern Virginia into D.C., new things to try, and new people to meet. Usually, that all would add up to a major meltdown, tears, and days confined to bed. Surprisingly, that didn't happen. Instead, I felt more proud, excited, accepted, supported, energized, and alive than I have in a long time, along with the expected extreme exhaustion and grogginess.

I received countless notes of love and support in response to my online posts about my experience with CFS/ME and the #MillionsMissing campaign, I met with staff from both of my senators' offices and was able to discuss with them the sad state of affairs when it comes to funding for CFS/ME, and I participated in a good old-fashioned protest in the nation's capital. We stood up for ourselves and millions of others who were too sick to attend (and sent only their shoes in their place) in order to demand the necessary funding and support to finally figure out this nasty, chronic, incurable invisible illness. Sitting next to an old pair of heels that I never wear anymore, in a sea of shoes that are never worn anymore, listening to and reading the stories of others who are also in this fight for their lives was a moving experience that I will never forget.

My birthday hasn't been the happiest or best time of year for me since I became sick eight years ago. It's a glaring reminder that I've spent another year sick, at home, not working, not moving forward. It typically involves a lot of tears and some dramatic statements. This year, my birthday fell in the middle of the #MillionsMissing events, which turned out to be the best co-incidence that I've experienced in a long time. Instead of mulling over the previous year and everything that had gone wrong with my health, everything and everyone I missed, and the fact that there is still no definitive test or treatment for CFS/ME, my mind was focused on the present. I thought about everyone I had met, all the stories I had heard and read, all the amazing humans involved in this fight, and I felt incredibly proud of myself for joining their ranks.

I realized something I never knew about myself: that not only can I be, but that I want to be an activist. I want to fight the good fight for funding, testing, trials, treatment, and a cure for this plague that has irreparably changed my life. So that's where you'll find me from now on, both online and in person, advocating for CFS/ME patients until there is a cure.

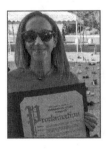

Tara A. is navigating life with chronic fatigue syndrome/myalgic encephalomyelitis (CFS/ME) and lives in Virginia with her husband and dog, Ellie. She loves to spend time with her friends and family, relax with Ellie, make jewelry, and enjoy as much time at the beach as possible.

Chronic Contradictions

WENDY KENNAR

Los Angeles, California, United States

I'VE BEEN LIVING WITH a chronic medical condition for six years now. It took about a year and a half for me to receive a diagnosis: undifferentiated connective tissue disease (UCTD). It's an autoimmune disease that has overlapping symptoms of lupus, rheumatoid arthritis, and myositis. I live with daily pain and fatigue in my legs, predominantly my left leg. Sometimes I feel as if I have weights strapped onto my left calf, making it difficult for me to walk. Other times, I feel as if my calf is being squeezed by a giant, evil set of pliers. Still other times, my legs feel heavy, as if some uninvited elephant has decided to plop right down on top of them. Even though my disease has been a part of my life for several years now, I don't feel as if I've reached a level of total acceptance and understanding. I am more and more convinced that living with a chronic illness is synonymous with living a life full of contradictions.

On the one hand, I'm thankful. Thankful that after a multitude of tests and scans, after meetings with various specialists, I wasn't diagnosed with anything fatal. Up until my autoimmune disease confirmation, I had been told that there were several possibilities: muscular dystrophy, cancer, leukemia, multiple sclerosis. Then a world-renowned rheumatologist handed me an alphabet-soup type diagnosis, and I felt like I could finally breathe. I would be around to watch my son grow up—he was three when I was diagnosed.

Flip that hand over, and you'll see there's another part of me that isn't thankful. I'm tired. Chronic means the pain goes on and on. This doesn't end. While many other medical conditions don't end either, some do. Some have treatments. Active things you can do to get yourself better, get yourself cured, and get yourself to the way you used to be. And the truth is, no matter how much I try to fight it or deny it, I will never be the way I used to be.

For the most part, my disease is invisible. I don't look like I'm suffering; it doesn't look like there's anything wrong with my body. In certain respects, I appreciate the invisibility factor. I don't have strangers asking me questions. I can blend in and make it seem like I'm the same Wendy I've always been.

But there are times when I feel like my life might be a little easier if my situation was a little worse. For instance, I was once crossing the street (in a marked crosswalk, with the green "walk" signal) in my neighborhood. My legs were tired that day, and admittedly, I was walking rather slowly. A driver was waiting for me to finish crossing before she could turn. She began tapping her steering wheel, looking at me, saying, "Come on, come on." She may not have thought about that incident any more after that, but I have on several occasions. It made my eyes fill up with tears, it made me feel badly that I couldn't finish crossing before the "don't walk" sign popped up. And it made me realize that if I had been crossing while using a walker or a cane, my slowness would have been more easily understood and maybe more readily accepted.

If my disease was visible, I might receive a level of protection, a bit more space around me if I was walking with a walker or cane. Now, when I try to navigate my son's schoolyard after the dismissal bell, I worry about my legs being accidentally bumped by a swinging backpack or lunch box. If I looked more disabled, less would be expected of me. I wouldn't be asked to volunteer to accompany my son and his class on their walking field trip. I have to say, "No, I can't chaperone," and hope I'm not asked why.

I want to be a woman who isn't defined by her disease. I want to go on living my life the way I always have. I want to go for walks in my neighborhood. I want to plan fun summer trips with my family. I want to do our family's weekly grocery shopping and take care of the household chores. I want to look at my disease and say, "Fuck you," as I take my son on a five-hour date to the Natural History Museum. I do that, but by pretending that nothing has changed, I'm denying a fundamental truth. Much has changed. I'm not as physically able to do those things. When I do, there's a strong chance my levels of pain and fatigue will increase. By admitting that there are things I can no longer do, I am also acknowledging a certain amount of loss and vulnerability.

I feel guilty for complaining about pain in my legs. It's pain, and this diagnosis has taught me that many people are, in fact, walking around with invisible pain. It's not just me. There are so many who have situations that are much worse than mine. There are people with no legs. So who am I to complain?

I am a mother and a former elementary school teacher. A woman who is used to explaining things to children, yet I still haven't figured out how to explain my autoimmune disease to my son. I have taught him what he needs to do to stay healthy and strong, to sleep, eat a variety of foods, drink plenty of milk and water, as well as exercise his body. I don't have the answers though when he asks me why I got sick, why my legs aren't as strong as Daddy's. I can't promise him that he—or other family members—won't get sick. I did all the right things, and I still got sick.

I am a writer, someone who considers herself proficient at expressing herself with words. Yet when asked, "How are you?" I am often at a loss for words. Many times, my answer doesn't change: "My leg hurts." But I get tired of saying it, and I assume that others (such as my husband) get tired of hearing it.

Especially when there's nothing anyone can do to ease the pain. So sometimes I try to gloss over the situation, answer with an ambiguous, "My leg hurts a bit, but I'm okay," but then I'm not being truly honest about how uncomfortable I really am.

Living with a chronic illness means there's a lot that's out of my control. I don't know how I'll wake up feeling. I don't know if it will be a good day or not. I don't know if a bike ride with my son will cause additional pain or if I'll finish the ride proud of what my legs can still accomplish. At the same time, there is so much to control while living with a chronic illness. I've got to stay on top of my medical appointments, follow up with the insurance company, take my medications on time, and refill my prescriptions. On a "good day," I walk around with surprise and gratitude and confusion. What's different about today that's making me feel so much better? What can I do to make this feeling last? Everyday tasks like emptying the dishwasher or watering the plants on my patio are suddenly so much easier. But on those same good days, a certain level of sadness creeps in as well. So this is what it feels like not to hurt? This is what I used to feel like all the time? Because until I have a good day, both my body and my mind have forgotten what it feels like not to have regular pain.

The word "chronic" is itself a contradiction. Chronic means long-lasting and persistent. In certain respects, those are good qualities to have. But when it comes to pain and illness, I'd rather it be temporary or occasional.

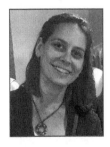 *Wendy Kennar is a mother, freelance writer, and former teacher. Her writing is largely inspired by her nine-year-old son and from the experiences of her twelve-year teaching career. Wendy's personal essays have appeared in a number of publications, both in print and online. You can read more from Wendy at www.wendykennar.com.*

Expecting Motherhood, Creating Self

SARAH MYERS

Chicago, Illinois, United States

WHEN I WAS THIRTEEN years old, I was told I'd never have children.

A group of doctors stood by my bedside as I woke up from anesthesia, murmuring in hushed voices to my mother. They'd just removed the ovarian cyst that had almost killed me. It had started to become infected, and my body had effectively shut down from it. But there was another problem. There were several more, large cysts. The doctors came to a consensus: I would never be a biological mother.

This is the part where all of my current friends get confused. "But Sarah," they say, "I thought you said you don't want kids!" Well, yes. That's certainly true now. I'm thirty-five, single, and far too broke to have children in my life. But when I was a little girl, I wanted other little girls. I daydreamed about a future where I'd marry Lindsey Buckingham (he was super cute in 1985, Google it!) and read our children *Pippi Longstocking.* I'd raise them to be sure of themselves, kind to others, and let them run around naked in the backyard until they were five or six. I'd sing them to sleep with Beatles songs or Disney, depending on my mood, and I'd dance with them in sunbeams. Most of us divorce ourselves from fantasy motherhood or fatherhood by simply being around children once we're grown up. Kids are cuter when you are a kid yourself. But I never had that chance. I was still a little girl myself, still playing with my American Girl doll Samantha and tucking her into her beautiful brass bed when I was told that having children would be impossible.

My own mother, to her credit, didn't tell the doctors they were horrible to their faces. Behind their backs, she swore and cursed them, telling me not to listen. "You've got a long time to figure out how to be a mom, if that's what you want," she said. But why want it? I'd just been told I couldn't have it. Something about how my ovaries didn't work right. Some defect in me that would make those lullabies impossible. I had been told my dream could never come true, so I set my sights elsewhere.

I became the friend that was good to talk to when you were down, the one that was always there with a hug and a harsh word for whoever had wronged you that day. I became good at nurturing sick folks, and I'm told that my soup has worked miracles. (Crush garlic into soup as hot as you dare make it, then crack an egg open on top for protein. Let the egg cook in the soup a little, then stir it in.) I became a mother of four-legged and two-legged creatures. I cluck to birds when I walk past trees, letting them know a large human is bumbling by so I don't startle them. I massage my oldest cat's hips, simply because he might be feeling his age by now. I know I like mine rubbed out, why not him? I am a mother, but not in the way that tiny Sarah ever planned. It's rewarding, but certainly not the path I'd thought I would take.

But, oh! There is another sad twist to the tale. Not only do my ovaries not function correctly—the left was so defective that doctors removed it when I was twenty-nine—I also have a disease called endometriosis. There are no benefits to endometriosis, just pain and more pain. It is also a leading cause of infertility. One day I was at the doctor's office, and I brought up the idea of having a hysterectomy. I thought that so long as I didn't need those parts, the parts that caused pain and could never give me babies, why not simply get rid of them?

"But what about kids? Don't you want them? You're so young, you'd be a great mother." The doctor smiled as he told me this, putting a hand over mine.

I don't think he understood why I burst into tears. I don't think I understood either. He retreated to the safety of the hallway, leaving me alone to mourn all the little hands—reaching up for mommy—that I will never be able to touch.

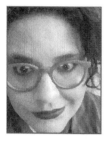

Sarah Myers is a graduate student studying thanatology. They hope to work with the LGBTQIA+ community as a grief counselor. In their spare time, they write, read, and watch more horror movies than strictly necessary.

Adventures in Snow Shoveling: January 9, 2016

DANIELLE LORENZ

Edmonton, Alberta, Canada

I'D SPENT THE LAST week cooped up inside as I was finishing the first draft of my candidacy proposal, so today, I decided, I would shovel some snow. For many of you this seems like an innocuous—and probably irritating—statement, as you shovel snow all the time (at least in the winter). Fair enough.

In terms of how around-the-house chores go, I don't mind shoveling snow. I like that it's a form of exercise. But I haven't been able to shovel snow in three years; this is to say I have been physically unable to shovel snow. It hurt far too much. This wasn't a "take a Tylenol" kind of pain. Tylenol stopped working for me following a surgery that screwed a metal plate into my ulna, which was by the end of my master's program. This was a "take prescription anti-inflammatories and get steroid injections" level of pain. Chronic pain.

Depending on how long you've known me—and the likelihood is that reading this, you don't know me at all—you may recall I had two major surgeries on my wrist in the span of a year. The first was a partial wrist fusion in December of 2013, where a set of medical staples was inserted between my wrist bones. The aim here was by decreasing range of motion by fifty percent, pain and inflammation would decrease. No dice. By the end of the recovery period I was in pain again. The kind of pain where I needed to take opioids to function.[2] I was desperate: I wanted to stop being in pain and finish my PhD. Again, surgery was my only option. Okay, fine.

In November of 2014, I had another metal plate screwed into my arm, this time attached to my metacarpals and ulna. It hurt. Like hell. I have never been in so much pain before. The prescription drugs they gave me were not effective the first two days. I had to stay overnight in the hospital after the surgery for the first night to get intravenous and oral meds. Following discharge on the second day, I had to go to the emergency room a few hours later to get an injection of morphine. That's how much pain I was in. It was hell. I wondered, "Is childbirth like this?" Anyway, the goal of this surgery was—after surviving the recovery process— decreasing the range of motion by 100 percent, meaning that if my wrist does not bend, my pain would stop.

Now that I'm fully healed a year later, my pain is better but not gone. I still take prescription anti-inflammatories, I still take Tylenol Arthritis three times a day, and in winter I still end up taking prescription pain killers as well. The assumption we're going with right now is that all the metal in my arm—two plates and fourteen screws—is just too much for my body to handle because my bone structure is rather small. At some point, this means I'll need an eighth major surgery to take it all out.

Anyway, back to shoveling.

Like most graduate students, I don't have a car, but I did have a car shovel and an empty space that my building required me to clear. I had the idea that if it hurt I was going to stop. Listen to

---

2 I say 'function' here loosely because you don't really function. You're mostly awake, but in terms of being able to do fairly normal, day-to-day things, it's like trying to swim through pudding. You end up being a gelatinous blob because everything is exhausting between being in pain, and the pain medications that make you drowsy.

my body and all that. So I bundled up and went outside. I noticed how light the snow was; it was that fine, icy stuff, rather than the heavy packing snow I'm used to from living in Ontario, Canada. Even though I was using a glorified children's shovel, since the snow was so light, shoveling was easy. I listened to my body and stopped when I felt it was time to stop.

I thought everything was going to be good. At most, a little sore from using muscles I hadn't used in some time, right? Wrong.

I became quite sore. It leveled off at the "good" kind of sore you get from a hard workout at the gym. This I can deal with. This I was at one point used to. However, my wrist hurt like hell. I have no idea what causes the wrist pain. It could be weather changes, pressure changes, precipitation, temperature extremes, how much I've used it, or the alignment of the stars. No idea.

The right side of my body—literally divided by my spine—had sore muscles. The wrist on the left side of my body hurt in a way that kind of felt like a broken bone. Additionally, my stomach hurt because I hadn't fed it enough; the prescription drugs have thinned out my stomach lining, and as such I produce more stomach acid which bores little holes if there's nothing in there to digest.

In the words of the great philosopher Homer Simpson, "You tried your best and you failed miserably. The lesson is, never try." Seems apt, no?

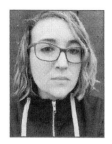

Danielle Lorenz is a PhD candidate in the Department of Educational Policy Studies at the University of Alberta in Edmonton, Alberta, Canada. Her academic work focuses primarily on how Indigenous and settler relationships manifest within Alberta's K-12 education system. Born with a congenital condition and developing others shortly after the onset of adulthood, Danielle's experiences as a chronically ill cis woman have affected how she sees herself within her scholarship as a settler on Indigenous lands.

I Am Not My Cornea

KEIDRA CHANEY
Chicago, Illinois, United States

IF YOU HAVE KNOWN me for longer than a day, or had a conversation with me that has lasted longer than twenty minutes, you've probably heard me talk about the fact that I am slowly losing my vision. Some people respond to such a reference with: "Oh yeah, I know what you mean. I wear glasses—I'm really nearsighted." I'm here to say that unless you have a disorder called keratoconus, no, you do not understand. Keratoconus is a disorder of the eye that causes changes in the shape and thickness of the cornea. This can cause blurry vision, double vision, light sensitivity, seeing multiple "ghost" images, and more.

So what does this mean for me, exactly? I've had keratoconus for about seven years. It has progressively gotten worse, to the point where I now need specially-fitted contact lenses in order to see. If I don't wear them, life for me involves seeing everything as multiple images of the same thing, blurrily overlaid on top of each other.

Reading is especially difficult. And, when working as a freelance writer and editor, that is a pretty essential skill. In the past four or five years, especially, my disorder has become a constant source of stress for me. One of the things that makes it hard is that my contact lenses are not gas-permeable, so they are prone to cause painful irritation and infection. Which means I have to take them out. Which means I can't see. My cornea has become so misshapen that I can't wear glasses anymore; when I do my eyesight still looks like multiple blurry images.

So the contacts are a must. I can't see without them. What's more, I am now prone to extreme, painful light sensitivity, which makes working in certain environments a major pain in the ass.

All that to say, I spend a lot of my time these days being hyper-aware of my environment: light, air pollution, and humidity all affect my ability to see. Sometimes I will do everything I possibly can for myself and still get an eye infection, and that really sucks.

I feel like I had a lot more fun, that I was a lot more fun four or five years ago when this wasn't a constant part of my daily life, mostly because I live with a lot of fear: What happens when my eyesight deteriorates to the point where the contacts don't work? What if surgery is so expensive it financially ruins me? What if I can't work for several months? What if there's nothing I can do in the future to revive my career if I stop working for a bit? What if no one is around who can help me when I finally get my surgery?

Even daily life and work bring a barrage of questions: What happens when I have an eye inflammation on a major deadline or meeting? What if people stop wanting to work with me if it happens too much? Do I tell people that I work with that I have this? If I tell them, will they see me as "damaged goods" and not want to work with me? When I worked in an office, I wondered, "Do I try to get accommodations in an office setting?" I work from home now, in part because of this issue. Will this be used against me if I bring it up? What if no one is around who can help me if I have a really bad inflammation and can't see? This has happened often.

I think about this last question all the time, mostly because I've had a couple of nightmare situations where I've been partially or completely blinded with no one around to help me out, and let me tell you, few things will make you feel as vulnerable as being stuck in a strange city or stressful situation where you can't see anything, your eyeballs feel like there are flaming-hot pokers beings shoved into them, and instead of people helping you see what's in front of you at that moment, they want to have a conversation with you about why you can't see.

But I get it, people don't know I'm having problems by just looking at me. For the most part, I can get around fairly well. I am not walking around with a cane. My eye problem is mostly invisible, except on bad days. But that's the frustration of it all. When I have bad days, it sometimes feels like I'm overreacting, or whining, even though when I am going through it, it really does feel that bad.

A major struggle is knowing that life as I knew it has changed, probably forever, but the new normal isn't stable enough for me to get used to it before it changes again. I still live in fear of losing my livelihood, because I know I can't operate as quickly or as precisely as I did pre-illness. I work in the especially fast-paced field of digital media, and I fear that I can no longer keep up.

On an up-note, I have learned a few beneficial things: the power of asking for help, which was very hard for me as a fiercely independent person, as well as the power of self-care. I get no extra points by pushing myself beyond my limits and if I don't speak up for myself, likely no one else will.

I've also become a lot more aware of the struggles of those of us with chronic and invisible medical conditions and disabilities. There are so many people who live and work with chronic illnesses and there's still so much shame around it. The narrative of illness is embraced largely when someone has "overcome" their illness or is cured. Many of us are never cured, and will live with our illness forever, but it doesn't make us less of who we are. I am still coming to terms with it, and it's difficult.

There's a story that keeps circulating about an Olympic athlete, Steve Holcomb, who has the same issue I do. It disrupted his life and he suffered from depression and suicidal ideation. I have too. But the telling of his story has been so focused around the cure that "saved" him and made him "whole" again. Many people with keratoconus have to live with the stressors of daily care for the rest of their lives. The cornea transplant may be rejected, the corneal thinning may return, and even after surgery you may still have to wear the irritation-prone lenses. Since the focus is on his "cure," it keeps things light, it makes the story more inspirational, but mostly for the people who aren't really going through this in the first place.

Even though I get sick of talking about my eye problem every day, I still do. Mostly I talk about it because it's my life, every day, and if you ask me how I'm doing, this is a big part of it. But I also discuss it because I see a lot more people with chronic medical conditions really making a point to not live in the shadows even as they are dealing with their illnesses.

There's this dichotomy about illness, a dangerous one that exists in our society, where you are either 100 percent well or 100 percent sick, and if you're sick, then you stay out of view until you're 100 percent well again, like Holcomb. And that's bullshit. A lot of us aren't 100 percent well, but we're fine, and we're living our lives as best we can. Rather than living a false life to make others feel better, we tackle it full on, knowing there will be good days, great days, bad days, and awful days, but through it all we are still ourselves. I am still me, and not defined by my keratoconus.

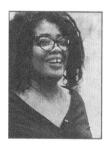 *Keidra Chaney is a writer and musician based in Chicago.*

PTSD: The Illness I Couldn't See

AMY OESTREICHER

Westport, Connecticut, United States

I GREW UP THINKING an illness was either a fever or croup. Illness was a stuffy nose, a sick day, just an excuse to miss a day of school. Then, at eighteen years old, illness took on an entirely different meaning. Illness suddenly meant waking up from a coma, learning that my stomach had exploded. I had no digestive system and I needed to be stabilized with intravenous (IV) nutrition until surgeons could figure out how to put me back together. Illness became a life forever out of my control, and a body I didn't recognize.

What my body experienced had no standard diagnosis. I needed ostomy bags and had gastrointestinal issues, but I didn't have Crohn's disease. Doctors were fighting to keep me alive, but I had no terminal disease. There was so much damage done to my esophagus that it had to be surgically diverted, but I had never been bulimic. I didn't fit into any category. I was just ill.

I became a surgical guinea pig: undergoing medical procedures, tests, and interventions. Devoted medical staff put hours into reconstructing and then re-reconstructing me, determined to give me a digestive system and a functional life. I eagerly awaited the day I'd be functional once again—the day I was finally fixed and back to normal. I desperately dreamed for the day I'd be discharged from the hospital. I'd be happy, healthy, and would finally know who I was again. Once I was physically back together, I'd be eating, drinking, walking, and feeling just like myself again. I'd feel real. I'd feel human. From there, I could do anything. Right?

Accepting Reality

After twenty-seven surgeries and six years unable to eat or drink, I came to understand that the body doesn't heal overnight. You don't wake up in the recovery room to a normal life. Stitches heal one by one. Neuropathic nerves grow back one millimeter a month. Learning to talk again took weeks. Learning to walk again took months. My skin's yellowish glare from the IV nutrition took years to fade. Not only was there no quick fix, there was no permanent fix either. I became accustomed to wounds reopening and leaking at any given moment; but with no other option, I learned how to accommodate and embrace my body for its resilience.

I was shocked at first and saddened that I could never get my old, unwounded body back. But what really surprised me was what had happened to my mind. Post-traumatic stress disorder (PTSD). I had never heard those letters put together before. I knew what physical trauma was, but I didn't know it could cause so much internal damage and disorder. I had a second illness, one that I couldn't see.

Discovering Post-Traumatic Stress

Not only had I woken up in a new body, but I also discovered a mind troubled with anxious thoughts, troubling associations, and upsetting memories. I was confused, and felt alienated from the rest of the world. I didn't understand I was suffering from PTSD until the internet explained it for me. The National Alliance for Mental Illness is an amazing resource with local chapters across the country. They helped me realize that I wasn't crazy. There were reasons why I was experiencing so many strange sensations. I was able to identify symptoms.

Intrusive Memories

People often ask me what the first food I tried was after the doctors gave me the go-ahead to start eating solid food again. After a few months of baby food, I was eager to dig right into my childhood favorites. I'll never forget that first French fry after all that time. I had been unable to eat or drink for years, and now that I was surgically reconstructed, the world was my endless buffet. I expected relief, fullness, and normalcy. Instead, I was jolted into a whirl of emotions. I was unprepared for flashbacks, images, and memories that I thought I had moved past. French fries became my trigger because putting food back into my body made me feel again. I felt everything: years of medical uncertainty, surgical intervention anxiety, and countless disappointments.

Intrusive memories became unavoidable. I would be sitting in a car and all of a sudden, I would start to panic. I felt locked in by the seat belt, restricted, confined, and unsafe. Suddenly, I was remembering what it felt like to be chained to IV poles, unable to move and constricted to a tiny space. My heart started beating rapidly and I started to panic as my memories intruded on what should be a perfectly calm moment. It wasn't that I was recalling a painful time. It was as if the doctors were right there with me in the car, peering over my open wound, dictating my uncertain future again.

Avoidance

I started to feel like I had to avoid any stimulant that might make me feel anything at all to avoid feeling bad. Nothing felt safe. I spent years locked in my room journaling for hours with my blinds shut, careful to block out any outside stimulation. I was afraid that if I had feelings, I might actually feel the deadliest sensation of all: hunger. I had been so used to avoiding my emotions in the hospital that all the feelings afterward were a tremendous struggle. I had grown comfortable staying numb. It was too painful to remember every setback and struggle, too overwhelming to recall everything I had lost with every surgery. I felt that I had lost my innocence, my old body, and even my sense of self, and I was doing everything I could to avoid confronting that.

Dissociation

When trauma left me emotionally and physically wounded, I disassociated to protect myself. I became numb so I didn't have to re-experience what had happened to me. This made my world a blurry haze. I would walk around as if a zombie, mindlessly pacing hallways and walking in circles, doing anything to keep my feet moving rather than my thoughts. I would tell myself things like:

- If I don't keep moving, I will feel awful emotions.
- I cannot pause to look at anything. If I do, I'll remember awful things.
- I must keep doing something, and I must always know what I am doing.
- I will be nervous if I am in a small space.
- When I feel pain, it is because I am in surgery again.
- I cannot stop moving. If I do, I'll drown.
- If I go outside I will feel too much and it will hurt.

Hypervigilance

I was extremely anxious and irritable. If I couldn't constantly fidget or find another way to numb my thoughts, I would panic. I'd become overwhelmed with intrusive memories and raw emotions. I misdirected my anger around the circumstances onto others. I couldn't sit still in classes and couldn't function as a responsible adult. These things controlled my life.

Owning My Trauma and Learning to Cope

My life changed when my stomach exploded ten years ago. PTSD is something I still struggle with because my traumas will always be a part of me. Despite all that has happened though, I've learned how to thrive. I've found healthy ways to deal with the memories, flashbacks, and emotions. For the first time, my life feels bigger than my past.

Healing didn't come all at once. For a while, every day I'd confront a memory a bit more. I called it "dipping my toes in" to my trauma. Finally, I could put words to my grief. I was able to write, "I am hurting." From there I had to befriend my past. Once I embraced my experience, I could tell my story. I let myself feel the pain, frustration, anger, and ultimately, gratitude. I could then speak to it. I gently taught myself how to live in the present moment, rather than be stuck in the world of trauma.

As soon as I wrote down words like sadness and pain, I could finally explore them. In time, I couldn't stop the words that flowed out of me. My memories started to empower me, and I wrote with feverish purpose. I would journal for hours as every memory appeared in my mind. Soon, the words weren't enough and I needed a bigger container. I turned to visual art. I filled pages with drawings of teardrops, lightning bolts, and broken hearts. Creativity became a lifeline, a release. Art was a way to express the things that were too overwhelming for words. The term for healthy PTSD coping skills is "self-soothing." Expression was my way of self-soothing.

The day I first shared my story with someone else, I realized I wasn't alone. There were others around me who had been through trauma and other life-shattering events. Being able to share my story emboldened me with a newfound strength, and the knowledge that terrible things happen. I found that if other people could bounce back, then so could I.

PTSD: The Mosaic I See

My perspective on illness has changed since I was a child, and it's also changed since my last surgical intervention. I've learned that illness isn't always present in physical scars. I've learned that some wounds aren't visible, and sometimes we don't even know we have them until we need to take care of them. I've also learned that I'm resilient and strong. I have been taken apart and put together again, differently, yet even more beautiful than before—like a mosaic. I'm still reassembling myself day by day and learning to love what I can build.

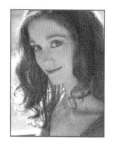

Amy Oestreicher is a PTSD peer-to-peer specialist, artist, writer, and health advocate. She's contributed to over seventy online and print publications, and her story has appeared on NBC's TODAY *and CBS. She is the creator behind the #LoveMyDetour campaign to help others cope in the face of unexpected events, which is the subject of her recently published memoir,* My Beautiful Detour: An Unthinkable Journey from Gutless to Grateful *(2019). Amy is a yogi, foodie, and general lover of life. Learn more: amyoes.com.*

An Echo Unheard

DEEPTI DILIP KUMAR

IAS Colony, Bangalore, India

"FIFTY-FOUR . . . FIFTY-FIVE . . . FIFTY-SIX . . . FIFTY-SEVEN . . ."
It sounds like the nurse at the station is reading someone's pulse, but she's merely handing out blue plastic tokens to the people milling around her desk. "Sixty. I'm sorry, ma'am . . . quota for the echo room's morning session is done . . . senior consultant cardiologist will begin his rounds shortly. Please take a seat and wait your turn."

She's skipping out words to save time and to calm agitated patients and their caregivers. I shake my head and leave my mother to it. I could tell everyone here it's futile to worry, to wait praying, to argue about appointments, and to bargain for an earlier spot. After thirty years of this routine, you kind of get used to it.

I shuffle back to the open hallway, fall into a steel chair with a slump, and play with a can of Diet Coke in my hand. The token, hastily tied to my wrist, says I am the fifty-seventh in line—the machine above my head beeps at number thirty-four and hasn't changed for twenty minutes now. There are twenty-three other patients awaiting their turn under the mysterious gaze of the echo wand. Who says I'm special?

My mother always said I was, and I had always accepted it as fact in my childhood. It took me almost twenty years, however, before I worked out *what* was different between myself and the other children in my class. Born with a congenital heart defect—that wasn't the special part, even if that was one in a thousand. Born with a rare, complicated physiology of the heart—that still didn't cut it, since surgeons and doctors had been making some headway into treating those types of defects in the decade that I was born. My speciality was that I was born in a backward, poorly-advanced country, where my chance of survival with this particular defect was close to nothing. Even assuming I had the right surgeries, which I did receive in a different country, my parents were playing with fate by bringing me up in this third-world hell-hole. In short, I was a miracle because of birth and circumstance combined.

Growing up in India was a struggle—for my parents more than myself. Indian schools are usually run privately, and strict about attendance. My mother had to find a way to explain my constant absences from school. They are usually strict about other apparently irrelevant things too—like whether you finish your lunch and participation in all the school's co-curricular activities. Many a time my mother had to come rescue me from an irate nun who demanded to know why I was taking so long over my lunch ("Why is she vomiting all the time?") and why I wasn't willing to run relay races for Sports Day like the other students.

It didn't take me long to realize there was a definite difference between myself and my friends, though on the surface everything seemed "normal." I couldn't muster up the energy to blow balloons for my own birthday party at age nine. I couldn't join in the marching band and drill sessions for Sports Day, and I definitely couldn't take part in the actual events themselves. My motor skills were weak and my coordination was terrible, so even simple games like dodgeball became frightening tasks for me. My handwriting did not stay constant throughout my schooling; there was a tremble in my hands because my arms didn't have muscle strength to grip a pen for long periods of time. When I was scolded by a teacher, or hit (which was common in primary school), my blood pressure would rise beyond all counts and I would faint silently, wetting myself in the process. Throughout the years, my mother pleaded with my teachers that I was a "delicate" child, but it fell on deaf ears. I didn't sit in a wheelchair. I didn't wear special devices. My mental development was similar to that of other students in my class. Since my disability was not apparent, I was given no special treatment. I was not a special child in India. I was just another child learning to adapt and be resilient.

A three-hour wait later, I am finally in the echo room. The technician waits for the senior consultant to join her, while two final-year bachelor of science interns stare goggle-eyed at me while I slip out of my bra in a quick motion and lie down with the gown covering my chest. The wand is slippery and the gel is cold. For half an hour, the technician and the doctor battle it out. They can't find what they are supposed to. "This heart looks totally different from a normal one," I hear the interns whisper. I catch shreds of phrases—ventricular septal defect (VSD), venous blood, lung capacity, Glenn shunt. I close my eyes and enjoy the coolness of the room and the soft murmur of the doctors' voices.

My father brought me up to love nature. As a result, trekking, or taking walks in the hillside, has always been something I thought I was meant for. The memory of me skipping beside my dad up and around hairpin bends was etched into my mind. We'd stop and smell the flowers, or pluck and taste the lemongrass. Often, he would haul his Nikon camera over his shoulders and bend down to photograph a butterfly or orchid. These memories made me love hill towns and their folks' easy cohabitation with nature. This March, however, I had let my walking group down. It was the first time I couldn't keep up with my friends. I thought I could. The hill was small, the incline was gentle, and my shoes were broken in. Yet, after ten minutes on the trail, I felt out of breath. My face filled with blood and itched. A pain, a searing pain, began in my jaw and reached my left chest. I sat down on the trail while my head splintered open. My chest was on fire and burning coals fell into my gut. That was the first sign of gradual heart failure.

My friends, who were not clued into the nature and extent of my disease, thought I was slowing them down, making it up, and causing drama on purpose. One of them led me back to the cabin. I leaned on his arm throughout the way down, waiting for the throbbing in my left side to stop. I slept that afternoon away and sat up that night crying. They didn't mention my defeat, but I knew I had failed them. I was a failure.

"A few instances of tachycardia, nothing unusual," the doctor says, smiling as he looks over my file. "Since your last visit, you're looking so much better. You've put on all the weight you lost from tuberculosis (TB). I am glad to see you looking cheerful again."

"She's been through a lot," my mother agrees. "Constant heart monitoring, now TB, now weight loss, anemia."

"She should be proud she's a survivor."

I smile but I do it with some difficulty. If I'm a survivor, why do I feel small and insignificant every day? Why do I feel like my life before me, my future, is like a black cloud in the distance waiting to burst over my head?

I don't want to say it out loud, but I know I'm depressed about the person I am and the situation I'm in.

The year I contracted TB was a difficult one. Not only did my grandmother die, my romantic relationship was broken off for good, too. Not because either of us had cheated, not because we meant nothing to each other anymore, not because of the distance. It was because he could not bear to think that he may lose me one day.

The first time I heard him say that, I laughed. Laughed outright. "You won't lose me!" I cried in amusement. But he had done his research, he said. He had downloaded PDFs, read academic data, spoken to a cardiologist he knew—the prognosis was slim. In fact, it was a miracle I had survived this far into it with no extra surgeries or treatment, especially given that I lived in a country where resources for both those options were woefully inadequate. I had no health insurance, no life insurance; the policies available to me were not valid to those with pre-existing conditions.

He listed about sixty-seven such reasons while my hand holding the phone went cold and I breathed in a rattled, TB-ridden breath.

He was not wrong. I went online and found friends with the same defect, roughly around my age. Some had fared well and some had fared badly. But I saw a pattern in all their stories—I was the truly lucky one. No extra intervention, no surgeries, no transplant lists, not even a single hospitalization in all the twenty-seven years after. Maybe I was truly special after all.

I tell the doctor, point-blank, with my mother in the same room, that I feel like shit. I feel worthless. Like all this "survival" has come to nothing. He seems concerned. "Aren't you enjoying what you do? You teach children, don't you?"

"Yes," I admit. "I love the children. But no one, not the kids, not my colleagues, knows the physical toll it takes on me."

The doctor puts his hands together and thinks. "Hmm," he says at length. "It's a tough situation. I have never felt the need to point out any risks or alarm you or your family, simply because your positivity all these years has been your wall of immunity. Of course you will find things difficult, you are quite different. What exactly troubles you?"

"This country doesn't have space for someone like me," I spit. "I have to put in nine hours of work a day too, I don't get benefits, I don't get any leeway. Being an adult here is tough but being a silent struggler here is worse." I am filled with anger and bitterness.

The doctor smiles sympathetically. "I understand. But look at those children out there, turning blue, trying to breathe. They fight for survival. You should look at the larger picture instead of focusing on day-to-day irritations."

"Children?"

"All the babies who were with you in the echo room. They deserve to know their fight is worth something. That their fight is valued and respected. You as an adult survivor lead them and give them inspiration."

This doesn't seem fair to me. No one is cheerleading me, no one seems to want to inspire me. I try to see the point he makes. As we exit the room, a newborn baby in a stroller coughs up phlegm and cries heartily, his lips and little hands blue with effort. My mother stops to tap his chin affectionately and smile at the nervous parents.

"Do you feel sorry for him?" I ask my mother almost jealously.

"No," she says simply. "He'll make it through."

I raise my eyebrows at her and she shrugs.

"Well, *you* were that little baby once." She sweeps out of the hospital, her head held high, her arms clutching the reports that are my actual life story.

Single ventricle, VSD, slight tachycardia, lung function compromised twenty percent, heart function compromised forty percent.

I follow her out feeling alive again.

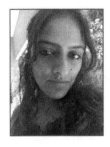

Deepti Dilip Kumar is a school teacher by day and writer, reader, and dreamer by night. While teaching children is her passion, she loves to study more about history, sociology, and the intersections between psychology and teaching. She enjoys fiction that deals with the new generation and their voice, and is particularly interested in journeys, both inward and personal, as well as outward and exploratory in nature.

Part 3

The Medical Side:
Diagnosis, Treatment,
Doctors, & Hospitals

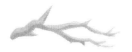

Pain

HERON GREENESMITH

Boston, Massachusetts, United States

A NEUTRAL SCENE: I walk with a friend, perhaps from class to class in college, across the spring-soft grass of the quad. My left hip aches and I slip into a limp, flinching from the hurt. My jaw is tight, clenched in pain and in anticipation of the inevitable.

"Are you okay?"

"I'm good, just a little twinge."

"Did something happen?"

"Oh no, just the usual connective tissue thing, joint pain messed-up-ness."

As the words leave my mouth, I cringe from their inadequacy. I cringe from my uncooperative hip and my uncooperative mouth. I cringe from my physical self, peeling away from the inside of my skin and muscles and joints, leaving my legs and arms fumbling as I huddle deep inside. Safe. Sure.

❖ ❖ ❖

I have chronic pain. I didn't rebel in high school, but my body did. As we—my body and I—grew into our fuller selves, lengthening, strengthening, curving, and straightening, my joints began to ache. My shoulders and hips. My knees and my lower back. My wrists and elbows.

✿✿✿

I have lived eighteen years with pain, holding pain, making room for it in my body, cherishing it. Never noticing its absence—pain is like that—and always noticing its return.

A diagnosis is, like any label, a privilege granted by the labeler. Labels carry power and control. The difference between medical diagnoses and other labels is that one cannot officially diagnose oneself. For example, I can label my sexuality—and that gives me privilege. I can name myself "bisexual" and most people will understand what I mean by that, even if I can't precisely articulate the various intricacies of my personal sexuality. The label is the shorthand.

Medical diagnoses, on the other hand, are labels you can rarely claim for yourself. Social norms and insurance regulations have created a structure in which medical diagnoses are on/off switches: you have or you have not. Our reliance on diagnoses makes it difficult for people without a diagnosis to legitimize their medical experiences—to get appropriate care, for example. The lack of a diagnosis by a medical professional can lead to the assumption that a medical condition isn't real, that it's psychosomatic or hysteria.

Receiving a diagnosis creates legitimacy. A diagnosis is the key to accessing appropriate and necessary care. A diagnosis is the key to gaining the understanding of one's peers, all of whom speak that same language of medical labels and share the same reliance on diagnoses.

A diagnosis is a privilege because not everyone can access appropriate diagnoses. Barriers to diagnoses and care are myriad: financial ability to access an appropriate professional; geographic proximity; ability to articulate one's symptoms, whether because of a language barrier or because of the nature of the medical issue; trust that you will be shown the courtesy and respect you deserve; knowledge that you *can* access a diagnosis and thus receive appropriate care; sexism; racism; homophobia; transphobia; ableism.

※ ※ ※

When my pain first surfaced, my mother was one of the few who believed me. She took me to pediatric orthopedists and hematologists across New England. At the orthopedist, I lay on the table in a thin hospital robe as the doctor squeezed my knees until I winced with pain. I retreated into myself.

"Does that hurt?"

"Yes."

I didn't wipe away the tears. I was relieved: people don't cry if they're not really in pain, right? So I'm not faking it, right?

The doctor was chatty. I answered his questions about high school with forced good humor. My mother was silent, leaning forward over her knees, watching me. Her face was tense.

The bone scan showed nothing. The thyroid scan showed nothing. The blood tests showed nothing. The echocardiogram showed my aorta at the wide end of normal and from there the crumbs of a meager diagnosis were scraped together from my various and disparate symptoms: mild potential connective tissue disorder, possibly Marfan syndrome. Recommendation: naproxen for joint pain, yearly echocardiograms for heart. Monitor condition.

※ ※ ※

I was young, I'm female, and my pain would ebb and grow and pierce and disappear. I lacked the authority of age, I lacked the medical vocabulary, and I lacked the concrete symptoms necessary for a hard diagnosis. Pressure is painful to my joints, but also along my ribcage and on my shoulders. Inactivity cramps my hips but excessive activity can aggravate my lower back.

Frustrated doctors listened to my inadequate words, looked at and inside my body, took the pieces of information they learned, and sewed together a story that seemed to fit, albeit clumsily. I couldn't articulate exactly when or where or why it hurt, so perhaps I was exaggerating.

Their doubt fed my doubt. I grew less sure of myself. Maybe I was exaggerating.

❁ ❁ ❁

The doctors were not alone in their assumptions. My first year with physical soreness was also emotionally achy. I found it impossible to fully explain what I was feeling. My father, hoping to ease my discomfort, would massage my shoulders painfully. When I asked him to stop, I could see his confusion and his own frustration at not being able to help me. He insisted on massaging my shoulders, his one response to his daughter's pain. I sat through the pain, unwilling to hurt him, even if it meant my own hurt. I thought that perhaps my pain was less than his, or maybe my pain wasn't real. And so my "no" slid away from meaning "no."

Chronic pain becomes a solitary experience. My world would color reddish black at the edges, but I knew that no one's world was tinged the same. I used my face to share my pain. Twisting the edge of my mouth. Gritting my teeth. Closing my eyes. Hoping someone would notice. Praying no one would notice.

❁ ❁ ❁

I have health insurance now, another privilege. And a primary care physician who listened to my medical history and offered me pain medication. I tried my unreliable "no." She recommended I go to the Marfan clinic at Johns Hopkins University to test my long-ago, far-away, semi-diagnosis. I said "yes," and I went, and I do not have Marfan syndrome. Nor do I have any connective tissue disorder.

I felt oddly complacent, distant from this news/not-news. Fifteen years of doubting, flinching, and never trusting myself or others had prepared me for this moment: there is nothing wrong with me and it was all in my head. The doctors were correct. My family was correct. The doubt overwhelmed me.

My primary care physician said, "I can prescribe you a pain killer."

"No."

"You probably have fibromyalgia."

"I really don't want to have fibromyalgia."

"You should see a rheumatologist."

❉ ❉ ❉

I was afraid that taking medication for my pain would further blur the edges between what my body felt—the electric twinges and dull throbs—and what my interactions with other people told me I was experiencing—nothing. I was terrified I would lose what little certainty I had, that my sharpness, physical and mental, would be rubbed away into a muzzy haze.

My pain was the only indication that I had pain. Only looking back can I try to articulate my deepest fear: that if I erased my pain, I would never be able to prove it existed.

❉ ❉ ❉

I improved at articulating my pain. It was an important process for my partner and I; he would become frustrated at my general aches and pains, my winces and sharp breaths, my inadequate mumblings. I was forced to find the words for what I was feeling at that moment—both to help him find a solution for the pain, like sitting for a moment or icing my hip, and to help me listen more closely to my body.

And by listening to my body and trying to articulating precisely what I was feeling, I knew that the pain in my hips, which had been slowly increasing over two years sending sharp stabs into my lower back, meant that something had to happen, some solution needed to be found.

※ ※ ※

My rheumatologist is a small thin woman with cold thin hands. I made the appointment at my doctor's urging. I had prepared for my appointment, sketched the history of my pain, but I felt a foreboding, a sense that this was my last chance. I worried that if she had no answers, I would not go seeking again.

The rheumatologist listened to me, without speaking, until I ran out of things to say. She then asked me questions about when my pain started and when it flared up. I struggled to remember, to articulate. With her prompting, I slowly painted the picture of my pain. She took off my shoes, looked at my feet, and pressed her cold fingers to my arches. Stood me up, looked at my knees and my back. She gently bent my hips and asked me to push my arms against her palms.

She sat back.

"You have high arches and hypermobility and your joints have been struggling for fifteen years to hold your body together. Your muscles are tight from cramping around your joints to protect them.

"No more flip flops. Arch support all the time. We'll get you a physical therapist to work out those tight muscles and you should do some core strength training. You'll never be better, you'll never be pain-free, but we'll get you well on your way."

Sometime later I was on the street, walking toward work. I called my mother. I started crying. Someone believed me. No;

someone believed my body. She could hear what my body was saying without me having to translate it into my too-often inadequate language. She could hear what my body was saying and she believed it. She believed it and knew how to start making it better.

❖ ❖ ❖

It has been four years since someone listened to my body, told me what it was saying, gave me the language to tell others, and helped me begin to fix myself. My pain has not disappeared—it never will. It has shifted, shrunk, sometimes sharpened. I have become infinitely better at listening to my body. I have become stronger. I have changed my life: only closed-toe shoes now, with arch support inserts. No standing for hours at a party. No popping one hip out when I stand. No crossing my legs at the knee now, only ankle over ankle, demurely, or ankle over knee, brazenly. I lift weights and do Pilates. And after, ibuprofen. Heat. Ice. Daily stretching and strengthening, lying on the living room carpet, coaxing my hips to soften.

With my diagnosis, I feel more confident asserting my pain. I let myself admit weakness. I can't walk five miles anymore. I sometimes need to stand up after sitting for hours during a meeting. I have a lumbar bolster on my chair at work. Before my diagnosis, I was afraid to explain myself in my own words, my own inadequate labels, those names that no one knew. Now I have my diagnosis to protect me, to privilege me. I also have the responsibility to protect myself by listening to my body and serving its needs. Now that I know what's wrong, I cannot ignore it.

My life stretches out before me, still filled with pain, but maybe also filling back up with trust. The process of learning to listen to myself has helped me listen to others and helped me speak to others. My partner has been with me on this journey and has protected me when I needed comfort and pushed me when I wallowed in self-pity.

There may be a community lesson here, a lesson I hope to learn: believe others when they speak. Trust when someone articulates a problem. Trust when they can't articulate it well. Use their words, not your own. Validate others' lived experience. Remember your own pain.

Remember your pain.

✲ ✲ ✲

A neutral scene: I walk with a friend, perhaps to get a sandwich at lunch, across the bumpy cobbles of back-street Boston. My left hip aches and I stop for a moment, clenching into the pain as I was taught. The spasm passes. My friend has stopped a few feet ahead.

"Are you okay?"

"Will be. Let's walk a little slower."

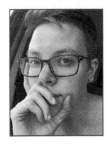

By day, Heron Greenesmith is a policy attorney for LGBTQ+ people. By night, they write fairy tales and do crosswords in between episodes of murder mysteries. They live with their little family in Boston, Massachusetts.

Going to the Emergency Department with a Chronic Illness

R.S. NASH

Melbourne, Victoria, Australia

WITH POSTURAL ORTHOSTATIC TACHYCARDIA syndrome, a form of dysautonomia, I often visit the emergency department for intravenous fluids. When you first arrive, you tell the triage nurse why you are there and give your medical history. Sounds simple, right? From the moment you mention chronic illness, they tend to treat you differently. They often don't know the condition well, and don't like the fact that you know more about it than they do.

When you come in nauseous, you'll need to try and explain that you have already tried anti-nausea medications such as ondansetron, but they don't work because of your condition. Recently when I told a triage nurse this, she nodded and walked off, coming back a few minutes later to tell me, "We are going to give you some ondansetron and see if that helps."

This, I find, is the biggest issue in the way emergency departments handle chronic illnesses: miscommunication and an unwillingness to learn. Whether they like it or not, doctors need to understand that the chronic illness patient probably knows

83

more about their body and what treatment is needed than they do, as this person has likely been here countless times before. It is immensely tedious when the doctors insist on doing tests to try and work out the cause of your issues when you have already informed them of what it is.

Doctors also need to understand that we deserve the same amount of respect and care as any other patient. If we end up in your hospital, you can be damn sure that it must be important, because we experience medical horrors every day that others would normally run to doctors for, and we just carry on with our day.

The last time I went to the emergency room, I was in the waiting room for four hours watching people with sprained fingers get seen long before me. I shut my eyes and prayed that when I did get through, the doctor might be unlike all the others I have experienced; and she was. Young and new to the profession, she was warm, and her body language didn't change when I told her I was there because of a chronic illness. She sat down and had a conversation with me, listening to what I had to say about my illnesses and what treatment had been helpful in these situations in the past. She did not run wasteful tests, or ignore my previous experiences, but rather went ahead and gave me what I knew I needed. She may not have been the most experienced doctor, and may have hit a muscle when inserting the intravenous line, but she was the best emergency doctor I have come across. She even put a note on my file at the hospital so that the next time I must go in there will be evidence of successful prior treatment.

Miscommunication and lack of understanding are driving a wedge between the emergency health care system and chronic illness sufferers. I praise God for that one doctor, and implore others to follow in her footsteps. Do not disregard a patient because they have a chronic illness. Listen to what treatments patients say have been effective in the past.

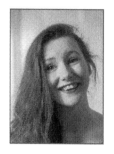

R.S. Nash is a twenty-year-old from Australia living with multiple chronic conditions. She likes to advocate and raise awareness through art and writing, and is passionate about helping reduce stigmas surrounding chronic illnesses.

Miss Treated

KATHERINE ERNST
Cheltenham, Pennsylvania, United States

"YOU'RE PROBABLY ANXIOUS."

"Maybe you're depressed."

"It's normal for nineteen-year-old girls to pass out."

I heard these and many more dismissive comments from virtually every doctor I visited when I complained of my symptoms: fatigue, recurring rash, joint pain, racing heart rate, and intermittent passing out. I now know that I have lupus, but it took about a dozen years and a lot of heartache to get to that diagnosis.

I went for years wondering if I was the hypochondriac they told me I was. I felt like a happy, motivated person. I thought I wanted to get out of bed when I physically couldn't do it. But what if they're right, I wondered to myself while I laid in bed for the third day in a row. I think I'm excited about the projects I'm working on. I really wanted to go out with my friends last night. But what if I'm so crazy that I don't even know that I'm crazy?

I finally went to see a psychiatrist, and I explained that my primary doctor had diagnosed me with panic attacks and depression a few years prior.

"Do you feel sad?" the psychiatrist asked me.

"Not really," I said. "I mean, I don't like it when I feel sick, but when I'm feeling well, I'm a happy person."

At this point in my life I was in my first year of law school, and I was not experiencing a flare. I felt well. I went out with friends weekly, and I was doing awesome in my classes—nearly straight As.

"What are your symptoms when you have these 'panic attacks'?"

"My heart beats very quickly sometimes," I said, "and it's uncomfortable."

"What do you do when this happens?"

"I sit down because I know it'll end eventually. It's disconcerting, but I try to ignore it until it goes away."

"Do you feel panicked at all?"

"No. It's happened so often, I'm used to it, so I just lay down and wait until it's over."

"You're not having panic attacks," the psychiatrist said. "That's nonsense, and don't ever let a doctor diagnose you with something you don't have again. You're clearly having some sort of cardiac issue and you need to see a cardiologist about it."

This was both the most empowering moment in my medical saga and one of the most deflating. On one hand, I was so grateful that a medical professional—a psychiatrist—was telling me that this wasn't all in my head. I didn't have an anxiety problem; there was something physically wrong with me. On the other hand, I was getting yelled at for believing a doctor when he'd made a diagnosis. What does it mean to say that I shouldn't have let a doctor diagnose me with something I didn't have? Aren't they supposed to be the experts on figuring out what something was? I'd finally come across a doctor who validated the idea that a medical diagnosis can be seriously flawed, and yet somehow he had still managed to find a way to make the other doctor's mistake my fault.

But why were so many doctors convinced that my medical ailment was something I was making up or that it was all in my head? Maybe I'm a particularly crazy-seeming person. I find this difficult to believe given all I've accomplished: graduating top of my class in law school, practicing law, writing numerous novels. No one outside of a doctor's office has ever accused me of being lazy or anything other than sane. In general, people view me as a highly competent person who is, if anything, overly fastidious.

I started talking to other women with chronic illnesses, and I heard the same story over and over. They went to the doctor and their symptoms were dismissed. In fact, I've never met a woman with a chronic illness who hasn't been accused of making up her symptoms for attention, having anxiety or depression, or being a hypochondriac.

I investigated it further and found it takes people with autoimmune disorders an average of five years and five doctors before they receive a diagnosis. Why? Because studies have shown that doctors commonly attribute women's symptoms of physical illness to psychological problems. Women die because of this every year, ranging from women who are suffering heart attacks being turned away from emergency rooms without even being tested because doctors assume they're just anxious, to women who die of brain cancer because doctors are quicker to chalk up their neurological symptoms to attention-seeking behavior.

I wish that someone would have told me back then that it's just not normal for nineteen-year-old girls to pass out. My symptoms were not in my head. I wasn't the crazy one—it's the medical community that's crazy. That's why I started the website Miss Treated. It catalogs the hundreds of studies showing that this sort of medical sexism exists and its blog is a place for women to share their stories of being dismissed by doctors so that we can all feel less alone.

That psychiatrist I saw all those years ago told me that I should never again let a doctor diagnose me with something I didn't have. That was harsh, but he was right. I now want to get that message out there to every other woman.

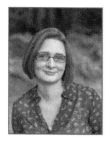

Katie Ernst is a writer and attorney who is passionate about the intersection of feminism and health care. Her website, Miss Treated, *collects stories of women who have been dismissed or demeaned by doctors. Follow her on twitter @MissKatieErnst.*

"...Sixteen, Seventeen, Eighteen..."

KATIE HIENER

New Milford, Connecticut, United States

"...AND THIS IS REALLY EMBARRASSING: Thursdays I wash all my hangers. It takes like three hours to take all my clothes off and set them on the bed just so. Then, I wash each hanger individually. After they dry I reverse the order that the clothes were originally in as I hang them up. I'm such a nutcase."

"You are not a 'nutcase,' Katie. As we've discussed, your obsessive-compulsive disorder has you in its grips at this point in time. Medication and talk therapy should see you to the other side. Obsessive-compulsive disorder (OCD) is no fun, certainly nothing you would choose. Unfortunately, your case is rather severe."

"But Dr. Benton, I mean how—why—did this happen? I can't do anything normally anymore. Everything I do entails checking and counting and cleaning and then more often than not, doing those things again and again. I'm tired. I hate my life and sometimes I wish I were brave enough to . . . well, you know."

"Katie, do you believe that you would hurt yourself?"

"No. My son would suffer and as a Catholic I don't want to rot in hell. I'm not suicidal, just tired. Sick and tired."

"I know. You just asked how this condition came to be. Unfortunately, we aren't 100 percent sure. It looks as if a combination of factors are the pieces of the puzzle: genetics, hormones, learned behaviors, and familial dysfunction. OCD is an anxiety disorder. Some people cope with anxiety by obsessing and acting compulsively. Last week, for example, you told me that your mother was an alcoholic and that she told you often that she wished you had never been born. That's powerful stuff, Katie."

"I can't fault her. She was a mess, probably due to the way she was raised. It just seems to trickle down, doesn't it? I mean, I'm terrified that this will happen to Jordon."

"You're not being asked to fault your mother, but to look at the ways in which she has caused you great distress. Jordon is a healthy, well-adjusted child who is being nurtured by you and Mark. It was wise and kind of you to have him take custody at this point. When Jordon spends time with you, you don't tend to act compulsively."

"True, but before our visits and after them, I'm a wreck."

"Would you rather delve into your family history some more, or role-play the cognitive thinking that we've been working on? You had quite a bit of trauma in your young life. Can you see that?"

"I guess so. Maybe I am hurt. Hurt or angry, I don't know."

"You can certainly feel both, and each is an acceptable way to react. Your challenge is to define your feelings, accept them, and then move away from obsessing. The medication that you recently started will take the edge off your anxiety. You'll be able to focus better and do the work you need to do here. So far, so good, Katie. Tell me about any rituals you have?"

"It takes me forever to brush my teeth. I count as I brush, and if the toothbrush slips or something, I have to start over from the beginning."

"Let's do this: before you brush, I'd like you to sit in a comfortable chair. Close your eyes and slowly concentrate on relaxing your neck and shoulders. Imagine that you are brushing your teeth. Brush one. Stop. Brush the next. Stop. Brush the next. Stop, and so on. Try your hardest not to give in to the temptation of counting or starting over. Each time those thoughts play out in your mind, imagine taking the brush away from your mouth, setting it down and leaving the bathroom."

"I'll try, but I'm not very optimistic."

"See you next week, Katie. Stay well."

Three years later:

"Hi, I'm Katie. I had a severe form of OCD for eleven years. Dr. Benton has asked me to sit in on your meetings as a client who knows all too well the struggle you're facing. Welcome everyone."

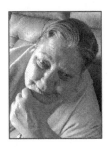

Katie Hiener loves playing with written words. Penning for online sites and magazines, Katie is also a storyteller, an animal welfare proponent, a psychology buff, and a connoisseur of fine pizza.

The Tale of a POTSie

BELLA

Youngstown, New York, United States

I'M BELLA, AND THIS is my story.

I am a college student who used to ski, sail, act, run, and play tennis, until I fell ill. It started a little over a year ago when I was in treatment for an eating disorder. I was experiencing symptoms for a while before I was diagnosed, but I thought it was my normal with anorexia. In the beginning of my treatment stay I was sent to the emergency room for very low oxygen levels, extremely high heart rate, and blood pressure that was bottoming out. After running a series of tests, I was released from the hospital the next day, diagnosed with what they said was a panic attack. I do suffer from anxiety and panic attacks as well, but the nursing staff and doctors at my treatment center were not convinced that my symptoms were due to my anxiety.

The next morning, when I was getting my daily vitals taken, things were still not looking good, and the nurse sent me back to the hospital. I was admitted and stayed for a week. In addition to being severely dehydrated, I was also diagnosed with postural orthostatic tachycardia syndrome (POTS). I received no recommendations for care and was released back to the treatment center to work on my eating disorder. The issues surrounding my eating disorder started to improve, but my physical health was declining fast. I was constantly dizzy and unsteady, and very fatigued. It reached the point where the doctors and nurses were putting me in a wheelchair just to get around.

When I was discharged from treatment, I came home with a walker and spent most days sleeping or lying in bed. My parents wanted to make sure that there was nothing else going on, so they sent me to the Cleveland Clinic. After my second tilt table test it was confirmed that I have dysautonomia/POTS with vasovagal syncope, and possibly autonomic neuropathy. This time, however, I got a care plan. I am still undergoing various tests to see if there might be anything else that I am suffering from, but for the first time in a while, I have hope.

Living with chronic illness has been anything but easy. It turned my life upside down. I was relieved, though, to finally receive a diagnosis, because I was beginning to think that I was crazy. I constantly thought that I was making everything up, and that there was nothing wrong with me. I would worry that I was a burden and my OCD had convinced me that I was a liar or a fake. There are plenty of downfalls that come with having a chronic illness, but in a strange way, I believe it really has made me a stronger person. And as much as my illnesses have been a curse, I truly believe that they may be a blessing in disguise. Sometimes it can be hard to stay positive, especially on difficult days. It did cause me to take a break from school for a while, and it is now taking double the amount of time to get my degree than it otherwise would have. I do try my best though, to stay positive, for both myself and my family.

One thing I wish my family understood, though, is that on hard days it is okay for me to feel discouraged, down, upset, or angry. Sometimes I feel like I need to hide or suppress my feelings when I am having a tough time dealing with everything because I don't want to seem like I am complaining or whining. I also do not want to make my parents feel even more helpless because I know there is nothing more they can do, and I do not expect any more from them. They are so supportive and have helped me tremendously. Sometimes, though, it can become exhausting trying to be positive all of the time. Sometimes I just want someone to sit with me while I cry and say, "I understand. It sucks that you are sick, and it's okay to be upset."

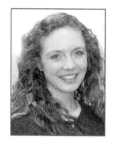

Bella is a graduate student studying social work, who is living with glycogen storage disease type XI, autonomic neuropathy, dysautonomia (POTS and vasovagal syncope), Raynaud's, and gastroesophageal reflux disease. She has a blog where she writes about living with these conditions, and she also contributes to The Mighty. *Her ultimate goal is to work as a social worker in a hospital setting. She would like to use her experience in dealing with chronic illness to help and support others suffering from acute and chronic disease.*

Chronic Illness Eugenics

CHAYA HAZEL CANINSKY

Boston, Massachusetts, United States

I'M SEVEN. MY BODY has been sucked into MRI tubes numerous times. I've been poked with needles and shocked with electricity in the name of finding a diagnosis I'm not sure I want. My spirit floats somewhere above all of this. Disembodied.

My neurologist diagnoses me with Charcot-Marie-Tooth disease (CMT). He tells my mom his reading of my DNA when I'm out of the room—a good call on his part, because understanding how to share hard information with children was definitely not part of his skill set.

I cry when I hear the news. It feels like my entire body has been labeled "different" and "wrong."

In a follow-up visit he warns me—at age seven or eight—that if I get pregnant it could make my CMT a lot worse. His words haunt me.

I don't know what to do with this information. I have no idea if I want to have children. But I definitely don't want somebody else making that choice for me. What would happen to my body if I had a child? What does "get worse" mean? The prediction is so nebulous. For the next several years that information hangs over my head like a stormy weather cloud.

In my teens I mention the pregnancy warning to the hotshot orthopedic surgeon I see for CMT. He tells me that he doesn't know of any medical evidence to suggest that pregnancy would affect my CMT. He tells me that all people who have a pre-existing condition tend to get a little more screening during pregnancy, but he doesn't think CMT poses any particular risks. I have more faith in his medical expertise than in the neurologist's. I feel relieved. I also feel really suspicious that my neurologist obfuscated the evidence to better accommodate his own prejudice the first time around.

In my late teens and early twenties I read Eli Clare's writing. I learn there is a theory called disability justice. There is disability community. And disability pride. Clare describes feeling shame when he is unable to climb a mountain. He describes unhelpful medical predictions and how he only narrowly missed being institutionalized as a kid. He describes learning to love his complicated body just like he learned to love his queer self. He found pride in his disability. He describes how complicated it all is. Suddenly, I feel less alone with my experiences. I write him an email and share too much—given we don't actually know each other—asking him how to find disability pride. He doesn't respond. I look elsewhere, hope ignited.

I start to understand that there is a widespread, often subconscious belief—held by pretty much everyone in our culture—that people who have disabilities are inferior.

At age twenty-two, I read *Undivided Rights: Women of Color Organizing for Reproductive Justice.* I learn how many actors in the United States have contributed to sterilizing, injecting with long-lasting birth control, and controlling the available social service resources of those whom the United States has always wanted to have disappear—Native Americans, disabled people, mentally-ill people, and poor people, among others. This history lives within me. It lives on in the disabled women I know. The history of exclusion and institutionalization lives deep in our bones.

We try to be perfect in order to be worthy enough to hold onto our place in human community. We are subconsciously aware there are many people who think that maybe it would be better if we were somewhere else, anywhere but here. No one says it aloud.

Our perfectionism and apologies have yet to succeed in rooting out the ableism that lives in the hearts and minds of our families and friends, in our schools and hospitals. Still, we apologize.

I come back to my neurologist. Neurologists are meant to read DNA like tea leaves—presenting the whispers of the future in case that might provide some meaning and context for the present. Some clarity for understanding our bodies and what interventions might be appropriate. They are not meant to be the gatekeepers of DNA. When they try to control my body or my friends' bodies and choices, they are abusing their power. This practice needs to end.

I love my disabled friends. I love my disabled body. There is no part of me that wishes to stop the replication of the DNA that created me or my friends or any of the disabled people who live in this world.

I recognize that it's complicated. In this world, some people have hordes of gold and some people have empty kitchen cupboards.

I live in the United States. I am a white, Jewish, class-comfortable, queer person. In school I had a physical therapist, speech therapist, and extra time to get to classes. I had the 504 law supporting my right to an equal education. I now qualify for jobs at which I can rely on my intellectual strength and not my muscle strength to secure the resources I need to make a life. I didn't get where I am alone. No one did.

I come back to my DNA and my decision regarding pregnancy. Every so often I wonder about my own decision to have children or not. I still haven't made up my mind. I don't want to pretend this is simple or easy. Disability has real consequences.

I think of my CMT as a variation—an experiment, a pilot project. Is the CMT combination of nucleotides an improvement on the design of muscles? Not really. But I also don't wish my CMT away. It is frequently inconvenient but not wrong or a defect. No, I view my stumbles as reminders to pay attention to my body, no longer as reminders of shame and otherness. My slower walking pace makes me pay more attention to the world around me.

The hubris of a neurologist who had met me three times and thought he should be an arbiter of my DNA shocks me a little. There is no one who knows the stories and potential of my DNA better than I do. And no one better equipped to make decisions about its replication.

I don't have the answer. But I do have a wish, or maybe it's a prayer: I wish for all children growing up with DNA variations to be welcomed into the world with lots of love and with no more fear than any other precious, vulnerable infant. I want them to have all the resources they need to survive and reshape the world for their own survival.

I want parents to not have to fear how that child's life will be made so much harder by the ableist world they are coming into. I want to not have to wonder if they will have the resources they need to care for a child with needs that are not already accounted for in schools, in children's clothing sections, in the medical equipment you can purchase cheaply at a pharmacy.

I want this for myself. I want this for all the potential parents considering their future possibilities.

And I want you, dear reader, wherever you are, whoever you are—I want you to love disabled bodies and minds. Because difference is not wrong. Variation is beautiful. And when we fit our variations together we get synergistic magic and community.

That is something everyone should have access to.

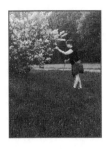

chaya hazel caninsky lives in Boston, MA. She works as a disability justice community organizer and hopes to get a herding dog soon. If this piece resonated or you have had similar experiences, feel free to share them with chaya at chayacaninsky@gmail.com. She likes reading reflections even though she often can't respond.

Pudendal Neuralgia

ATARA SCHIMMEL

Newton, Massachusetts, United States

I MISS YOU. I am still grieving for you. It has been three and a half years now since I lost you, and the grief is profound. It comes in cycles; I wish that it were linear. I wish that I could grieve and then move on. But my soul does not work that way. The sense of loss comes and goes. When I embrace what is left of my life and have a spiritual sense of belonging to my present life, I feel certain that I am moving forward. When the pain is sharper and when my body is incapacitated by exhaustion, the sense of loss hits again. Depression sets in and it is stubborn, as stubborn as the insomnia that has been my nightly partner ever since I began taking Cymbalta.

Before I started Cymbalta I was severely suicidal. Every night, when the pain moved beyond a level that my mind could bear, I cried and fell into despair. I believed that the only way out of the agony was up to me taking action. Euthanasia is not legal in Massachusetts, and all other forms of suicide other than swallowing pills terrified me. I had no idea what pills could do the job. I fantasized about poisonous mushrooms and about dying in the desert from heatstroke. I fantasized about starving to death in the forest. These were fantasies that I took comfort in. It was the thoughts of drowning myself, hanging myself, slitting my wrists, or jumping from tall buildings that took over my mind every night that terrified me.

Time becomes a profoundly subjective experience when one is suffering. My mind and body inhabited a reality that was completely separated from "normal reality." I knew that I inhabited a reality that no "normal" human could ever comprehend. The only people who understood where I was were those who were embodied by the very same beast. My body had been taken over by the devil. My body had become a torture cell; my body had become a curse that I was chained to. This hell had no reason and no God. There were only empty expanses of loss, despair, anguish, shock, and trauma that served no greater good and served neither God nor Goddess. There was the ever-present weight of suffocation. There was a full gamut of tortures: high voltage electric shocks, deep and relentless stabbings, wrenches twisting, razor blades slicing, and acid and fire burning through my vaginal flesh. There were bowling balls twisting my insides apart, bats jammed up my anus, and there was nausea and terror that accompanied all of these daily "experiences." If these sensations that my nerves were signaling to my brain had been due to physical attacks I would have been blessed with death after the first round. Instead, I suffered these tortures every evening knowing with certainty that the following evening would be just as excruciating.

Attacks of severe pain can be terrifying to witness. The eyes go back and forth at a frightening speed. One looks possessed; one feels possessed. Crying, screaming, pleading for death, banging your head against the wall, closing yourself up in closets, taking off all of your clothing, rocking yourself back and forth, and responding with terror when touched are examples of the many strange behaviors that I exhibited. When I was in severe pain the sensation of clothing on my body became unbearable, thus the need to strip naked. An innocent touch felt like stabbing erratic eye-movements—squinting and constant blinking were all responses to the pain I felt. The ring of the telephone frightened me and sent my heart racing. I was suffering from severe anxiety and deep depression. I struggled hard to maintain a sense of self and an identity. I felt as if I had become the pain.

I trudged my way to physical therapy twice a week. There were many sessions of internal and external trigger point injections. About eight months into physical therapy I started feeling relief. Menstruation would send the pain skyrocketing. But during the few weeks when my pain was lower I gathered strength, hope, and faith in my body's ability to heal. My caretakers recommended that I have Botox injected into my pelvic floor. I took their advice and trusted their assurance that the Botox could not cause more pain, but it sent me back to constant levels of excruciating pain. The progress that I had worked and suffered so much for was lost.

There were attacks of pain that were so strong I began splitting. When the pain was bearable, I was me. When the pain became unbearable, "She" was the one who experienced it. It was after one particularly cruel attack, where it felt as if a steaming block of cement had taken over my entire body, that I began splitting. After many hours of being stabbed deep into my vagina, morning arrived and the knives receded back into their sheaths. My body, spent and exhausted, fell asleep. When I later awoke I went to the toilet. On my way back to my room, my brother, who had spent time that night holding my hand, greeted me. I pointed to the blanket in the corner of my room and asked if he saw what happened. The blanket looked strange to me. It was not me that had been laying there. The body that was walking back into my room was a different one from the body that had been there that night. In that experience, I had become two separate entities.

It was summer. I rocked myself back and forth on the floor of my room. I cried to my doctor and to my therapist, explaining that I could not bear the levels of pain that I was in. I sobbed and spoke about suicide often. I was told that when the Botox wore off in six to eight months I would hopefully feel better. After the night of dissociation I told them that I could not bear another night like the one that I had just experienced. I was petrified. I begged for narcotics, begged for something to take home with me for if the pain was ever that strong again. They refused and I lost faith. After, I stared out of my bedroom window for three days. It was during that time that I promised Her that She would never go through another night like that. I promised Her that I would protect Her. This idea of someone else changed my views of suicide. It became my responsibility to protect Her. But it was also my/Her right to die. I/She deserved mercy. I figured out which pills would do the job and I knew how much I would have to swallow.

I woke up in a hospital bed with my mother on one side of the bed and my father on the other. They asked me if I knew where I was and if I knew why. I told them I did, I had attempted suicide.

Once it was clear that my liver had not suffered damage, I was transferred to the psychiatric unit. Cymbalta was added to the 300 mg of Lyrica that I had already been taking. Once the dosage of Cymbalta was titrated to the full 120 mg, the nightly tortures that left me pleading for death were gone. A few weeks later, I joined the Brigham and Women's Pain Clinic and met my new pain doctor, who understood the profound suffering her patients were experiencing. Though she's never physically felt what we have, she feels the depth of our anguish with the depth of her compassion. I finally began reconstructing my life, my identity, and my faith.

I feel a profound sense of responsibility to all the men and women that suffer and will suffer from pudendal neuralgia (PN). Childbirth, hysterectomies, prolonged sitting, bicycle riding, falling onto the pelvis, weightlifting, and exercise can all damage the pudendal nerve. My pudendal nerve suffered damage shortly after I joined a gym. I was taking aerobic exercise and aerobic kickboxing classes. My symptoms started deep inside my vagina, as if my cervix was being pinched and pulled by tweezers. For the first two years these symptoms came and went. I searched for help from different gynecologists who all prescribed yeast suppositories, or said the problem was in my head because my vagina looked healthy. I continued to exercise and to sit for lengthy periods of time, unaware I was damaging my pudendal nerve and causing the pain. It was after a long-distance flight that my symptoms began to intensify. Within six months I could no longer work, clean my house, or prepare food for myself. At the age of thirty-four I moved back into my parent's home.

Most gynecologists and primary care physicians do not know anything about PN because they are not taught about pudendal nerve damage in medical school. If the physicians I saw had learned of this condition or taken time to research it, I would have been told to stop exercising immediately and to avoid sitting for long periods of time. I could have potentially continued to live my life without any major disruption. Many pain doctors also do not know of the condition that is PN. They will recognize, though, the type of pain that the patient is describing as nerve pain. Unfortunately, pain doctors expect that their patients are exaggerating their pain levels because they are nefariously in search of narcotics. Consequently, many PN sufferers are under-medicated.

It may be too late for many of us to get diagnosed and treated before our injuries develop into chronic pain. But it is not too late for our children and grandchildren. We have the proof and can show our doctors what they need further education in. We need to demand that genital pain syndromes be a part of every medical school student's curriculum. Vaginal pain remains much in the land of "no research" and "no funding." How many more women will die and how many will live to tell stories like mine before we realize that the change will only come from us? Shame and privacy is fueling the suffering that we so desperately need to end. I send out a cry to all of us who are afflicted by genital pain syndromes: do whatever you can do to create awareness in the medical world and in the general population.

I pray to see the day when doctors will demand an education in pain management. I pray to see the day when general medical school curricula are revised to include research and information about chronic nerve pain conditions. Gynecologists and urologists must learn how to diagnose and treat vaginal and penile pain that is nerve and muscle related. The American Congress of Obstetricians and Gynecologists must create guidelines, educational objectives, and curricula for PN. Millions of women and men will continue to suffer as desperately and needlessly as I have if this change does not happen. From knowing how excruciating and traumatizing nerve pain is, I pray to be able to give voice and visibility to our suffering so that we will be received with compassion and care by doctors, family, friends, and community.

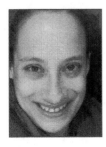

Atara Schimmel can be found painting, singing, and writing poetry. She is a lover of nature, finding solace with the animals and by the ocean. She continues to heal herself through creative expression daily.

The Monster Within

ANNIE WITTENBERG

Greensboro, North Carolina, United States

THE GYMNASIUM FEELS COLD and dark. The walls are so tall and the ceiling is so high that only giants could reach it. The sounds of four-year-olds echo in glee; their musical cheers bounce off the metal walls of the gymnasium in waves of harmonious noise. Colorful bouncy balls jump around the gymnasium almost as excitedly as the little bodies that fill the room. This flutter of movement and enthusiasm is a typical day in kindergarten. An outsider looking in would see a sea of children, smiling and laughing. Joyful souls celebrating their favorite part of the school day: play time. Fourteen children immersed in their games while child number fifteen sits on the sidelines feeling the cold tile beneath her and butterflies in her stomach. Child number fifteen was me.

Since I was four years old, I can remember feeling the jitters in my stomach, sweaty palms, and a general discomfort participating in novel activities. I only felt safe watching my classmates from a distance; putting even a foot out to join their rambunctious games would be too risky. Even when my gym and homeroom teacher tried to coax me into joining the other kids, I would defiantly refuse. I wasn't a defiant child, at least no more than any other developing four year old, but there was something that was different about me.

Years later, I would learn the name of the monster that held such a tight grip over my mind and body. The monster that would keep me lying awake at night worrying about what might happen the next day at school, what could be the next uncomfortable situation that I would find myself feeling trapped and suffocated in. This monster would trigger nausea, racing thoughts, and general feelings of panic. I carefully planned to avoid certain people and situations that made the monster scream out inside my head, "Too much! Too much! Let's get out of here!" This monster's name is anxiety, formally known as generalized anxiety disorder of the chronic variety.

I learned of the monster's name when I met with my first shrink at eleven years old. The diagnosis process went quickly: I filled out a few psychological questionnaires and answered some questions, all the while annoyed that her office smelled too strongly of peppermint and incense. Then, voilà! I was officially labeled as an anxious child. Once the monster had a real name, I hoped it would shrink away and disappear. I was sadly mistaken. Unfortunately for me, the gymnasium experience was just the beginning of what would become a crippling disorder. As I grew older, my anxiety grew, too. It became more intense and prolonged in its duration.

When I was six years old, my brother John was born. His birth was both exciting and anxiety-provoking, as the emergence of a new sibling typically is. Three years later, when I was nine years old, John was diagnosed with autism. He was fairly low-functioning at that time, and the chaos that consumed my house was distressing. John's outbursts, my mother's tears of frustration, and my father's consuming depression sent my anxiety into overdrive. I couldn't fall asleep, stay asleep, eat properly, or feel comfortable at home or at school.

That may be one of the worst parts of anxiety: when it grips you so tightly that there is no safe, calm place to retreat from it. I remember my third grade teacher pulling me aside and asking me, "What is going on? What's wrong, Annie?" At nine years old, it's still hard to explain the grip of anxiety and its toll on your existence to yourself, much less to another person.

I had my first panic attack in sixth grade. I remember it very clearly; I was in the cafeteria, which was crowded and noisy with my sixth-grade classmates as usual. The combination of noise, the mission of finding a seat where I could blend in, and the food that made my stomach queasy would rev up my anxiety each and every day of middle school. I honestly don't know what set off the panic that day, but very suddenly—like a gust of wind knocking me down and sucking the breath right out of me—I felt it. My hands started shaking and I began hyperventilating. I looked around at all the faces, I could see mouths moving but I couldn't understand the words. It felt like someone had pressed pause, and then fast forward. Everything was fuzzy and moving too quickly. Tears started pouring out of my eyes uncontrollably and my breathing became elevated. The kids at my table turned and stared. The girl next to me was saying something to me, but I couldn't understand her. I wanted to run out of the cafeteria but I felt tethered to my seat. It was a horrific feeling that can only be described as sheer panic.

The girl beside me led me to the teacher table in the middle of the room. The short walk to the table felt like I was being dragged through thick mud. I tried to block out what I believed to be every pair of sixth-grade eyes burning holes in the back of my head with judgment and confusion at the sight of my melt-down. My homeroom teacher asked the girl to take me to the of-fice. None of the adults seemed to understand that I was having a panic attack any more than I did.

The walk to the office distinctly stands out in my mind. The phrase that kept replaying in my head suddenly poured out of my mouth and I repeated it over and over like a broken tape re-corder: "I want to die. I want to die. I want to die." I said it over and over like a mantra or a prayer. It wasn't true: I didn't want to die. What I wanted was the tsunami that was drowning my body with fear and stress to stop. I wanted the mental and physical anguish to stop.

After the incident, I started meeting with a really good therapist. She was pretty and young. She spoke softly and her tone and body language were inviting. I answered her questions without much hesitation. She told me something that I still think about now as a twenty-two-year-old woman.

She told me, "Annie, all those thoughts in your head, those are racing thoughts. Racing thoughts happen when you have one thought that makes you feel anxious and then that thought spirals into another anxious thought and so on and so on until you feel stuck and unable to get out of your racing thought brain."

Whoa! I thought. This was the "aha" moment that I had so desperately needed without even knowing that I needed it. Not only did my therapist validate my thoughts and feelings, but she really understood what was going on inside my head. In that moment, I felt hopeful. Someone else in this world gets it. Maybe things will get better.

And things did. I am better. I still have racing thoughts every single day, I still have times when I'm so anxious that I panic and feel like I am suffocating, and I still have times when I become paralyzed and can't move for hours. The main difference between my experiences with anxiety as a child compared to now, though, is that I have a language that I can use to acknowledge what is happening inside my head and body during my anxious times. I have built a support network of compassionate people I can rely on to help me through those anxious moments when my toolbox of coping skills just isn't enough to help me self-regulate. These changes in how I cope with my chronic anxiety make all the difference when it comes to my quality of life.

The content of my racing thoughts has also shifted as I've aged. When I was ending my final semester of college, my racing thoughts swirled with new questions. Questions such as, what if you don't graduate in the spring? What if you don't graduate with a 4.0 GPA? You have to graduate with a 4.0. Oh shit, what if you do get a 4.0 GPA, but they forget to denote your name on the graduation ceremony pamphlet? Oh god, next weekend, traveling to Miller's graduation, what happens if you get lost and the GPS fails? Then you're late to the ceremony and disappoint the family.

Despite having racing thoughts like these, I've learned from various therapists and medical professionals how to understand key aspects of them as well as how to counteract them. An anxiety specialist pointed out to me that the common thread woven into all my racing thoughts is the phrase, "What if?". What if X, Y, and Z does or doesn't happen? These what-if thoughts lead to a slippery slope of worrying about future events that could happen but may or may not actually happen. Usually, my what-if thoughts lead me to picture a catastrophic ending that is very unlikely to happen, and instead blows the whole worry far out of proportion.

Sure, there's a chance that I could be late to my cousin Miller's graduation due to my poor sense of direction and the GPS failing. These obstacles could lead to a catastrophic ending of my family being upset. The chances of that actually happening, though, are very small. It only feels very large and probable when the what-if thoughts start flowing. My racing what-if thoughts lead me to constantly worry about future events, and this takes away from my ability to be present in the moment. Once I understood this, I became more mindful of when my racing thoughts begin, and I can then shut them down and return to the present moment.

One way I redirect my racing thoughts is by imagining picking up a remote, and pressing pause on the thoughts. I then ask myself an important question, "What bad thing is happening right now?" This question, which I learned from my brilliant anxiety specialist, has helped me through countless racing thought traps. The answer always boils down to, "Nothing. Nothing bad is happening right now. I just feel anxious." I'm not trapped in a fire,

I'm not in danger, my racing thoughts are just making me feel like I am. And yes, these thoughts and feelings are uncomfortable, but realizing that nothing bad is actually happening provides a huge sense of relief and the chance to return to the present moment.

So here's what I know: anxiety will almost definitely be a part of my daily experience for the rest of my life. And that sucks, because anxiety is uncomfortable. But I also know that I am not powerless when it comes to dealing with this monster. I have the tools, I have the strength, and I have the support to deal with anxiety as it comes. My anxiety has shaped me into being a more compassionate, empathetic person. It has taught me to be aware that many people have their own monster inside, be it anxiety or other chronic mental health issues. I feel hopeful about my life. The monster is there, but I have the power to put him back inside his cage when he emerges, and I can be free of him.

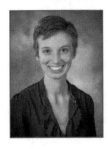

Annie Wittenberg lives in Greensboro, North Carolina, where she is currently earning her master's degree in clinical mental health counseling. As a future counselor, Annie hopes to support and empower people who are battling chronic mental health conditions. Annie finds daily joy in cuddling her sweet puppy, May, connecting with friends and family, and spending time outside.

Part 4

Acceptance:
For Better or Worse

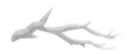

Good Morning

KAITLYN M. SMITH

Gray, Tennessee, United States

EVERY DAY IS THE same. You wake up, a process a lot harder than it should be. There are two alarms set on the dresser across the room so you can't turn them off in your sleep. You still end up hitting snooze multiple times, and have slept through them before anyway. The snooze button's extra nine minutes is never enough. The hour nap is never enough. The eight hours, twelve hours, sixteen hours of sleep you got last night is never enough. You feel like you could sleep for a week and it's never enough. You even tried sleeping through a whole weekend once, but it just left you aching, and still exhausted.

When you finally wake up, you wonder if it's worth it. When every day is a fight, you wonder if today is the day that you stop caring. The day you quit your job, drop out of school, and just stop fighting. Sure, that would come with all sorts of unnameable and horrible consequences, socially and financially, but you're not thinking of that right now. You're thinking of the pain in your abdomen and the pain in your head and the fuzz of exhaustion in your brain. You're thinking of the spike of pain that's coming when you stand up, you're thinking of stumbling off the walls to get to the bathroom. You're thinking of dealing with your coworkers or dealing with your classmates and of having to be awake and functional for eight hours, but mostly you're thinking of how nice it'd be to curl back up and sleep.

But today is not the day you give up. Instead, you stumble into the bathroom and try to get ready as best you can. More than likely you forget to brush your teeth, or hair, or both. You go to pick your clothes, and as soon as you touch a shirt your hand jerks away—not that one, not today. The material is too rough, or it's too tight, or it's too cold, and you need to pick your armor based on your daily weaknesses. So, on the ugly shirt goes, because pain does not give you time for fashion. You thank the powers above that you don't have to do anything that requires dressing up today. The dress shoes are enough to make you cry.

Next are the stairs, arguably the worst part of your morning. You grip the rail and the wall on the other side, and make your way down a painful step at a time. Your joints click with each step, and you need to walk with your legs twisted sideways to avoid relying on your knees too much. You reach the bottom of your daily Mount Everest, and sigh. Another small victory won. Now to determine what to eat. Food is hard, and not just for the effort that goes into making it. As you stumble into the kitchen, you stare blearily at the fridge. All the food looks about as appetizing as eating dust. You open the cabinets, and wonder why you haven't gone grocery shopping to get breakfast food. You will later remember that it's because you haven't felt up to surviving the grocery store. By chance, your eyes pass the clock on the microwave, and you nearly jump out of your skin. You're going to be late again if you don't make up your mind.

You grab the nearest to-go food (some rolls—hopefully enough to keep you going until lunch) and stumble to the door. You shove your tennis shoes on. They aren't the prettiest things, beaten up and dingy, but they're what you've got as well as being the only thing to not make your feet hurt. Next goes on the sweater, probably unnecessary for the weather, but it's your sensory security blanket. You take a deep breath and stop for a moment. Your pain is no better. Your hips feel like they're made of fire, the pain in your knees radiates down your shins. Your abdomen is full of burning acid and knives. You're so exhausted you could fall over. You stop, and you think: this would kill anyone else. This would keep anyone else home and in bed all day. This would have anyone else running to the doctor.

But you are not anyone else. You are you, and you have a life to keep trying to live. You exhale, and open the door.

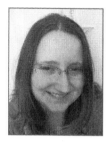

Kaitlyn M. Smith is a recent psychology graduate currently working in mental health case management. She lives with two cats, a husband, and way too many plants. In her free time, she enjoys writing a little bit of everything—including fantasy, poetry, and narratives about life with chronic illness.

Snakes & Accessibility Ramps

ALIX PENN
London, United Kingdom

WHEN I WAS SEVENTEEN I went on a school trip to Greece. It
was a fantastic trip, eight days of classical study, visiting muse-
ums, and splitting into small groups in the evenings to visit clubs.
I'm a massive nerd, and spending a week solely studying English,
classics, and history was utter perfection. We explored fishing
ports, saw the Acropolis, and investigated traditional hole-in-
the-wall restaurants. I was with friends, traveling somewhere
that I had never been before, and doing something I loved.

It also marked the first time I used a walking aid for an extended length of time.

We still don't know what exactly provoked my chronic pain
condition; although having been diagnosed with Ehlers-Danlos
syndrome (EDS) has pointed me in the right direction, doctors are still baffled. Before this trip I had used wheelchairs and
crutches for short periods of time when needed, but I clung desperately to the semblance that I was independently mobile. But I
wanted to make the most of the trip, which I knew would involve
a lot of walking and a higher level of mobility than I was able
to perform alone. Common sense won out. I bought a walking
stick. Even with it I fainted from pain and exhaustion more than

once, had to rest in the middle of the day while my friends took a guided walking tour, and developed welts on the inside of my palm from the weight required just to stay upright. Regardless, I would do that trip again in a heartbeat.

While visiting the ruins of an Asclepeion, an ancient healing temple, my teacher told me in a serious tone to sit out part of the tour and they would come and get me afterward. Perplexed, I did this. I sat on the steps of an ancient Greek temple and took photos, listened to my iPod and waited twenty minutes or so. Afterward they told me there was some concern that our guide— whether out of humor, benevolence, or mischief—had been talking about pushing me in the snake pit to "cure" me. I don't know how much of that was lost in translation, but the concern was real enough to stop me from going along with them.

No one has ever asked me if I would want a "cure." If a magic pill, an operation, or even if being pushed into a pit full of vipers would work, no one has asked if I would take it. And to be honest, I don't know. My chronic illness and chronic pain conditions have become so intertwined with my identity that I wouldn't know who I was if I were able-bodied. I was once able-bodied; I was a healthy and happy child who had only ever taken time off school once after an intense glandular fever. Then suddenly, one day when I was twelve, I was in so much pain I couldn't walk.

You develop a lot as a person in your tweens and subsequent teenage years. And I lost all of that momentum in one fell swoop. I can say with certainty that I would be a completely different person had I not grown up disabled, and more specifically, had I not grown up chronically ill. There is an obvious tenacity to chronic illness, and refusal from your body to improve. After eleven years of physio and hydrotherapy, hospital visits, pills, intensive treatments, blood tests, and using a cane, I am more mobile than I once was and am persevering. But I am not and never will be "cured."

My body is wired incorrectly, my nerves have mutated beyond "normal" comprehension; however you describe it, I will never be able to return to the pre-chronic illness able-bodied state. Do I want to? On the one hand, yes—desperately. I would love to wake up without pain. I would love to be spontaneous and not have to plan for consequences days, weeks, or months in advance. I'd love to be able to wear heeled shoes without the risk of dislocating my ankles, and I'd love to be able to sleep at night without the agonizing distraction of the pain that simply lying down causes.

But, on the other hand, if you were to take away my chronic pain, not only would the last eleven years of my life suddenly not make sense, but a huge part of my identity would be stripped from me. I'm involved in disability activism and I see the world through "the social model." I subscribe to an identity politics school of thought where Spoon Theory[3] is so entwined in my life that friends send literal spoons to show they're thinking of me. I don't know who I would be without this disability. The way that I not only see my future but also view my past is colored through a haze of chronic pain.

Sometimes it makes me sad that I can't remember what it feels like to not be in pain. Sometimes the thought that I can't remember and will never again experience something that so many people take for granted is so upsetting that I sit and cry. But more often, that lack of a tangible memory, a memory gap of what "able-bodied" means, is a blessing. I can see it, I can witness my peers and friends do things that I can't without serious repercussions, but I don't feel it. It's like trying to invent a new color. I don't have the capacity for it, let alone the ability to articulate what it means. I simply do not know what not being in pain feels like; my life has settled into this new normal.

---

3 Spoon Theory is a concept developed by Christine Miserandino and fully explained on her website at butyoudontlooksick.com. "Spoons" is often used as shorthand for the available capacity to manage fatigue and other symptoms of chronic illness.

I've got a new walking stick now. I wore the other one away and replaced it. I need to replace the replacement soon. No matter how sturdy something is, if you use it every day of your life it starts to wear out. That's a little like the human body in general, especially when you have a chronic condition. It's rather poetic when you think about it. My palms no longer blister from the stick; instead, the skin has become tough. It's uncomfortable, but it works. My life in five words.

I still don't know the answer to that question. The one about being thrown into the snake pit as a cure. It's certainly something to think about.

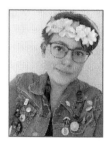

Alix is a stereotypical geek focused on history, musical theatre, and disability activism. She's lived with chronic pain and disability for over twelve years, and resides in London with a dog, six fish, and a walking stick.

Anxiety Is My Constant Companion

DEVIN REYNOLDS

Cedar Falls, Iowa, United States

I STILL FIND IT shocking when I talk to someone that doesn't really believe in mental illness. Having grown up in a small and conservative community, there was a large portion of my own life where I found the idea of mental illnesses confusing. I was raised with the unspoken belief that "where there's a will, there's a way" and that anything you put your mind to could be accomplished. So it didn't make sense to me that someone's own mind could hold them back. I always figured it was due to a lack of willpower on their part. In retrospect, the truth seems obvious to me. After all, the brain is an organ like any other, a physical object that can be damaged. A person's energy and willpower at first seem like ethereal, intangible concepts, but they are almost literally a result of how much of a particular chemical is in their body. Unfortunately, I didn't learn this until I was in my final year of college.

At the time, it felt like I was going insane. I couldn't stop worrying about every event in my life, from work and tests, to even casual conversations with friends. It felt as if doom was lurking behind every corner. No matter how much I told myself that there was nothing to worry about, it was like there was a voice in the back of my head that I couldn't silence. A voice telling me that everything was going to fall apart, no one loved me, and I was going to lose my job, drop out of school, become homeless, and die in a gutter somewhere.

I started to have trouble sleeping, and I was tired all day and night. I couldn't concentrate in school or at work. My grades were slipping fast; I used to be a straight-A student, and now I was getting Cs and Ds in every class. My relationships with friends and family were falling apart, and my performance at work was suffering dramatically. I reacted to every stressful event with uncontrollable fear and anger. I didn't know what was happening. I knew something was wrong with me, but mental illness didn't cross my mind at first. I thought maybe it was a flaw in my character, that I was doing something wrong, or that I just wasn't trying hard enough.

I don't remember what first made me think of mental illness, but once I did, I was desperate for answers. For the first couple years I was a true cyberchondriac—I must have diagnosed myself with twenty different disorders. I thought I was depressed, then thought I was bipolar, then thought I had obsessive-compulsive disorder. At some point I even thought I might be schizophrenic.

My friends urged me to see a therapist, but I resisted. As a child, I had gone to a therapist for anger issues, but instead of learning how to deal with my anger I only learned how to internalize it and bottle it up. I didn't trust psychiatrists or therapists; I thought they would just make me worse. And perhaps I thought that seeing a psychiatrist would be admitting defeat. I didn't want to admit that I was broken because I still thought it was just a matter of willpower, of forcing my brain to work correctly.

But it didn't work correctly. I nearly dropped out of college. I switched jobs every ten months. I ended a six-year relationship with my girlfriend. I was at the end of my rope. It really hit home when, after barely managing to graduate, I asked for a letter of recommendation from my favorite professor and he wouldn't write me one because I had done so poorly in his class.

Finally, I decided to see a psychiatrist. It wasn't an easy decision, and in some ways it really did feel as if I was giving up. But at that point, I felt like I had nothing else to lose. I was surprised by how good it felt to finally just let it all out. It felt incredible to hear my psychiatrist say the words, "generalized anxiety disorder." It gave my demon a name; it made my mental illness somehow more real, more tangible.

To tell the truth, it never really stopped being difficult—it only became more manageable. Taking medication every day felt strange, and it felt unnatural to rely on chemicals just to keep my brain functioning properly. Even then, it wasn't like my symptoms disappeared. They were less severe, but the anxiety was always there in the back of mind, especially on the most stressful days.

Even after getting used to taking my medication, I still have panic attacks—albeit less frequently—and sometimes it's difficult to work and make friends. Deep down, I still don't have much confidence in myself. I may never be able to have a well-paying career like my parents do, such as working full time at a hospital or becoming an engineer. I have more strength now though, and I feel like I can pursue my dream of becoming an author.

I will never be cured, but denying my illness, or trying to "defeat" it, will only ever do more harm than good. I wanted desperately to be normal, but that only left me more vulnerable. My mental illness will always be a part of me, but once I learned to work with my illness instead of against it, I was able to regain control of my life. When I felt a panic attack coming, my natural response was to try to ignore it or prevent it from happening, and this only prolonged the problem. When I acknowledge it and let my brain work through the issues naturally, I can greatly reduce the severity of my attacks and recover faster. It wasn't easy to realize this; it is largely thanks to my medication and the sessions with my therapist. Anxiety is my constant companion. I can never get rid of it, but if work with it, I can become stronger.

If you're dealing with anxiety, I know how hard it can be. But I promise you, if you seek out help, and accept anxiety as a natural part of your life, you can still live a fulfilling life.

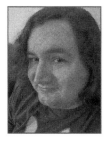

Devin Reynolds lives in northeast Iowa with two roommates and three ornery cats. He dabbles in video game design and is working on a full-length fantasy novel.

What Is It Like?

HANNAH REMBRANDT

Uniondale, New York, United States

I'VE GOTTEN A LOT of questions about being ill. But no one has ever asked me what it's like. No healthy person has ever wanted to sit down and really hear how bad it is to have chronic pain. I don't blame them for this—it makes sense. Why would anyone want to hear how horrible their friend, family member, or acquaintance feels? But it makes me wonder what I'd say if someone ever did ask.

It's hard, I'd say. It's hard on so many levels.

There's the obvious one: the pain. Having to go about my daily routine with the feeling of someone digging a shovel into my back, or having the desire to just cut off my arm because that would probably hurt less. But that's just the tip of the iceberg.

It's hard having to wake up and know that you can't wash your hair that day because you don't have the strength in your arms to hold them above your head for that long. It's hard to have to use way too much energy (that you really didn't have in the first place) just to leave your room because the door is so heavy, so much heavier than it was yesterday. And you have to have your high-arm-pain-day bras, because there are some days that reaching behind you to do or undo the clasp is impossible. The days when you can't wear the shoes you want to because you can't bend your back to pull up the zipper or tie the laces.

It's hard to know that no matter how many doctors you see, no matter how many medicines you take, the pain is never really going to go away. It's hard knowing that there is no cure. It's hard knowing that without a miracle of some kind you are going to have another seventy or eighty years of pain and suffering. Because that's the only way this pain is going to leave and never come back: a miracle or death.

It's hard to know that you're not yet twenty and you have the ailing health of an old woman. That you make jokes about your fibro-fog-induced idiocy and your arthritic fingers that make you take longer on your tests, and make you not able to sew even though it's the only thing that calms you down sometimes, but the jokes sound hollow to your own ears.

It's hard when no one realizes that your smiles aren't always real. It's hard when no one notices that your smiles aren't present. It's harder when they do notice and they ask you what's wrong and you tell them you're just tired because of course you're tired, but not the way they think. It's hard because you're tired of smiling when you don't feel happy, and people you know, people who care about you, ask you what's wrong even though it's the same thing that's always wrong. And it's hard when you realize that at least for that moment they forgot about your illness, and it's hard when you realize that you don't have that luxury.

It's hard to know that your friends won't ever be able to understand what it means to be ill. That no matter how much they love you and care about you and try to help, there is a gap of understanding that they just can't cross because they have never felt the kind of pain that you feel every moment, every day.

It's hard when you start to resent your friends for being able to do things that you'll never be able to do. You love them, and everything they are, and you start to hate yourself for resenting them because it's not their fault that they're healthy any more than it's your fault you're sick, but in your weak moments you just can't help yourself.

It's hard when you realize that all you want, all you really want, is for someone to sit down across from you, take your hand, and ask you what it's like and want to hear the brutal truth. All you want is for someone to recognize that you're living through hell every day and that you just keep living and that you are so strong for doing that.

It's hard when you realize that the hardest thing you have to do every day is survive.

And it's hard when you realize that no matter how hard surviving is, you're going to keep doing it for those seventy or eighty pain-filled years, because you are strong, and no amount of pain or loneliness is going to keep you down for long.

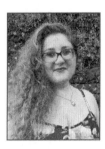 *Hannah is a graduate student studying speech-language pathology. She has fibromyalgia, rheumatoid arthritis, and lupus, and feels that these are an integral part of who she is and who she will become. Hannah looks forward to her future and is excited to be on the path she is currently on. Hannah is a generally happy person both because of and in spite of her illnesses.*

Forgive Yourself for Saying No

GLYNIS SCRIVENS

Brisbane, Queensland, Australia

DO YOU FIND IT hard to say no? I certainly do. Sometimes so much weighs on your answer that the temptation to say yes anyway is enormous. To hell with the consequences, we think, this is too important. Except consequences matter. Don't give up what you've worked so hard to regain. This is a lesson I have to learn and relearn regularly. Circumstances change but the central issue remains the same. I know I need to say no, but I feel it isn't acceptable.

Two of these "to hell with the consequences" moments presented themselves in 2014. Both times I agonized over whether it was possible to say yes. I was awake at night in the wee hours trying to find a compromise. I'll outline the circumstances and let you ask yourself what you would've done in my shoes.

In February, I received an invitation to a good friend's sixtieth birthday celebration. Liz and I have been mates since the 1970s. We have one of those relationships you can pick up at any time and find it's as good as ever. She probably doesn't understand my symptoms, but she knows me well enough to never feel any doubts about their veracity. The lovely card she sent was filled with little metallic "60s" that fell out of the envelope and sat on my dressing table for weeks. I didn't want to say no but didn't see how I could say yes.

You see, Liz lives in Canberra, and I'm in Brisbane, twelve hundred kilometers away. Her celebrations were a dinner party at a restaurant. I just wasn't up to it, but I desperately wanted to go. As the day was approaching, she sent a message. "Did you get the invite?" I'd messed about too long, unrealistically hoping my circumstances would change enough to let me go. They didn't. Reluctantly I explained that it was more than I could manage. And Liz was okay with that. "Don't worry," she said. "I'll come up and visit you." I'd turned myself inside out over this. I should've simply phoned and talked it over with her.

The second situation 2014 presented me with was even harder. What do you say when the stakes are high, and the other person doesn't understand your circumstances? When saying no will rebound and echo through your relationship in the years to come? What do you do then? I found out in July.

I received an invitation to my nephew's wedding, to be held in mid-October. The worst possible timing for me healthwise, as, for some reason, my body is always at its lowest then.

As details of the ceremony and reception emerged, it was obvious that it was way beyond my capabilities. The wedding venue was in a small village north of Melbourne in the middle of nowhere. This meant that even if I could somehow fly down early and rest beforehand, there'd be nowhere on that day for me to rest. The timing posed problems, with the wedding service at four o'clock and the reception beginning at seven o'clock. Guests would be standing around with pre-dinner drinks while the photographs were taken. All very well—if you can stand that long. I certainly can't.

Knowing all of this, I dithered, unable to say no. The reason? My nephew had a brain tumor. The most malignant type. His chances of survival were 3 percent. He was organizing a wedding while in the throes of a heavy chemo routine. I suppose I felt that

I ought to be somehow able to go the extra mile. After all, look at what he was going through. In the highly-charged emotional environment surrounding his wedding, saying no on the basis of poor health was not going to be understood. I realized that. And I knew if I was in his parents' position and unfamiliar with myalgic encephalomyelitis, I might not understand either. Difficult as it was to say no, I came to realize that nothing of value could be gained by my going. And much ground would be lost. I have my own needs and the needs of my family to consider.

What would you have done in my shoes? How would you feel about your decision? Would you feel compelled to accept the invitation, or would you put your own health first? It was a very difficult decision for me to make. What I did was ask my general practitioner's advice.

"Of course you can't go," Leanne said. "Why don't you try to spend a week in Melbourne when the weather's warmer? Meet your nephew and his fiancée for coffee. That way you can catch up with him properly. You wouldn't even see him, even if you could go to the wedding." So we made a plan. A compromise. It should've been my focus all along, but when the stakes are high, it's not easy to think clearly.

Consider these two situations. Compare them with the issues you face from time to time. And remember, never be afraid to look after yourself. There'll be times when, like me, you need to forgive yourself for saying no.

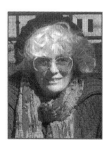

Glynis Scrivens is an Australian writer of short stories and magazine articles. Her book Edit is a Four-Letter Word *includes what she has learned about the writing process. Glynis lives in Brisbane, Queensland, Australia, with her family, two dogs, a Himalayan Persian called Mr. Floof, nine chickens, three ducks, and goldfish. She can be found at glynisscrivens.com.*

Forgive Yourself for Saying Yes

GLYNIS SCRIVENS

Brisbane, Queensland, Australia

ONE OF THE LESSONS myalgic encephalomyelitis has taught me is that sometimes I need to say "Yes," when I'd rather say "No, thank you." Is this something you need to learn too?

I always look to my grandmother's philosophy. She lived with us and helped my mother wherever she could. One job she always did was shelling peas (this was in the days before the frozen variety existed.) We needed to shell enough for eight people. She had arthritis in her hands and would ask for volunteers. Even when more than enough of us offered, there was always a space to sit. "Never turn back a willing helper," she'd say.

When I first became ill, and was bed bound, my children were very young. My youngest was only twenty-one months old. There was an enormous amount of housework needed to keep our family and home functioning. I was no longer able to do any of it. That was when I first learned to say yes. A friend from church kindly offered to come over to help. She had five children of her own, which made me hesitate. My mother reminded me of my grandmother's advice though, so I accepted Margaret's offer of help one day a week. The result was that our little family stayed afloat. With her help, and much support from my family as well, I was able to rest enough to begin to improve.

When I was well enough, I arranged for paid help once a week. A wonderful young woman named Lisa collected my children from school and cooked dinner every Friday. We had our groceries delivered every week, as well as fresh fruit and vegetables. Then my mother offered to pay for a cleaner. I'd already thought about this but decided I couldn't cope with a stranger in our home. Is this how you would feel?

Fate intervened. A young woman who did cleaning for our neighbor came to our door one day because she'd locked herself out. We instantly got along well, and soon she was coming to clean our place every Friday morning. This meant our weekend visitors were now greeted by a clean and welcoming home. You too may find the benefits of paying for a cleaner outweigh the loss of privacy. Don't dismiss the idea out of hand.

The years passed, and my children grew up. My health improved. And when my husband retired, we no longer felt we needed any external help. It was a reassuring feeling after so many years of dependency. Have you had one of these periods of remission? Did it last?

Our circumstances changed when I developed glandular fever four years ago. In an all too familiar scenario, the ground I'd gained healthwise was stripped away from me.

One doctor suggested a wheelchair. Once again, my pride stood in the way. But fate intervened again. Daniel O'Donnell, an Irish singer, was going to perform in Brisbane. I wasn't going to miss his concert, so we rented a wheelchair. We paid for a month, and made the most of it. My husband gallantly pushed me for kilometers as I rediscovered places I hadn't been in years—the city center, lovely walkways by the Brisbane River, parks, and shopping villages. I felt sad when it was time to return the wheelchair. One day we noticed a secondhand wheelchair for $140 and bought it. It's a real asset. We even take our young kelpie for walks with the chair, her lead attached to the handle. A sight that brings a smile to many as we go for our "chariot rides" by the river.

Recently, an even bigger decision arose—whether to install a stair lift. Something I'd never seriously considered, despite being unable to manage our back steps for years; thirteen steps that have stood between me and many activities. Glandular fever took away my ability to do basic things like using our laundry, which is downstairs. It also meant I could no longer feed our chickens or collect the eggs. Driving home from the shops one day, I noticed a woman in a nearby house gliding down her front steps and hopping into an electric scooter and zooming off. I felt envious. Why couldn't I do that too? Have you considered installing a stair lift?

I assumed it would be beyond our budget. Then there was the image. They're inevitably associated with infirmity, old age, and ill health. I didn't want my home to take on this image, and I didn't want that image myself. But when I watched this woman, words like infirm didn't cross my mind. What I saw was mobility and independence. Yet despite the evident benefits, it was an even bigger yes for me than the others. It took me seven months to pick up the phone and call a company for a quote.

Last Friday the stair lift was installed. The cost was $5,500; quite a bit less than I'd expected (and there was an option to pay by installments).

Why did I hesitate for so long? Concern that my children would worry about me, misplaced pride, financial concerns, on it goes. And I'll bet you've felt the same. What are the thoughts and feelings that prevent you from saying yes? Try to focus on the improved mobility these things can provide. Why lose opportunities to live a fuller life?

Remember my grandmother's advice. Never say no to a willing helper. When you can afford equipment that will improve your quality of life, just do it. Sometimes we need to say yes.

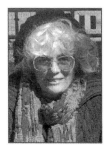

Glynis Scrivens is an Australian writer of short stories and magazine articles. Her book Edit is a Four-Letter Word *includes what she has learned about the writing process. Glynis lives in Brisbane, Queensland, Australia, with her family, two dogs, a Himalayan Persian called Mr. Floof, nine chickens, three ducks, and goldfish. She can be found at glynisscrivens.com.*

Grieving the Loss of Body

BRET STEPHENSON
Reno, Nevada, United States

I'VE BEEN GRIEVING THE loss of my body's health since I was twenty-seven, which is frustrating because I was in such good shape back then. My orthopedic surgeon told me I could not withstand any more injuries to my knees without serious surgery, so I bit the bullet and stopped competitive sports. I had always been an athlete, but that day, I felt the first death of activity in my life due to health. Shortly after that, my first back twinges started, and while I had more back pain than others my age, I held together pretty well until I was about forty.

I had survived Tahoe, Nevada winters for almost a decade. Snow removal then became increasingly painful. I slowly went from cutting, splitting, and stacking my firewood to buying the rounds and splitting them, to buying split cord wood, and finally just having the pile dumped on my driveway and paying a teen across the street to stack it for me while I stood feeling helpless and useless as a man.

When I use the term grieving, I am referring to Elisabeth Kübler-Ross's famous five-stage grief cycle we go through to fully process the loss of a loved one, a pet, a good job, children moving away, and countless other losses in life. I learned of this grief cycle, which is most associated with human death, when I got into adolescent counseling for a career. I quickly saw how to apply it to other forms of loss, including my health issues.

For those not familiar with the cycle, it is most easily remembered by its acronym "DABDA," with each letter standing for one stage of the cycle.

1. DENIAL: "No, it could not have happened; I don't believe..."

2. ANGER: Where we become angry that someone left us, that our marriage dissolved, that the good die young, that life is not fair, and so on. This is where many people get stuck on the cycle.

3. BARGAINING: Here we tend to try and bargain a better, usually impossible solution: "God, I'll do anything you want if you just bring her back..."

4. DEPRESSION: Once we fully realize the situation is not going to change, and we've spent our anger and begging for a miracle, it is common to get depressed over the loss. This is normal—you just don't want to get stuck here.

5. ACCEPTANCE: When we finally learn to live with the loss. Here we typically end up with that bittersweet, nostalgic feeling when we think of the loss and we're able to move forward.

My back continued its decline despite efforts to curb the problem in dozens of ways with thousands of dollars. I kept losing things I loved to do as they became either too painful or the after effects of the effort got me later. Through my forties and eventually after my first two back fusions at fifty, I began to grieve the loss of almost everything I used to find joy in. I sold or gave away all my Tahoe toys: golf clubs, snowshoes, tennis rackets, backpack, canoe, and eventually minor things like my last baseball mitt and football. I found myself unable to even play catch. Having my daughter when I was almost forty, I came to realize that I had never held her without pain, even as an infant just days old. Most recently I had to stop my passion of wood-working, which was also a way to supplement my income.

With each garage or eBay sale, my body demanded more time on the couch and soft chairs. I started refusing to go to restaurants and meetings, when I knew the seating would be painful today or tomorrow, often both. My income and passion for helping people with teens took a hit when travel got harder and harder. Soon I could not sleep in a normal hotel room. Driving more than a few hours was out of the question. I paid for more motels as I had to cut my drives into segments. Friends eventually stopped asking me to do things, and I began to feel like an albatross around everyone's neck, picking and choosing venues and situations I could adjust to, or usually, just tolerate.

All through this period I kept thinking about the grief cycle to help me cope with all the loss. I believe it helped me particularly with the anger and the depression. The cycle reminded me not to allow myself to stay stuck in any one stage for long if I could help it. I'll be honest, it wasn't always easy as the list of what I couldn't do soon fully eclipsed the list of things I could do.

More drugs for pain. Three fusions and more than twenty pieces of titanium turning my back into a half million-dollar Erector Set. Scopes, needles, MRIs, CT scans, X-rays, back braces, and canes became my new reality. I lost the ability to stay self-employed and had to revert to working for others. My evenings of writing books, teaching myself Photoshop and web design, and knocking down a master's degree all went by the wayside in favor of movies and distraction from being unable to get comfortable in any position.

My wife and daughter took walks without me and brought me food back from the restaurants they went to. Cooking, dishes, and other mundane chores began to hurt more and more. I hauled cushions everywhere I went because I didn't know what the seating would be like at any new spot. I stood over my wife, instructing her how to repair or adjust the sprinklers, fix the rain gutters, and a hundred other guy-chores that ate at my pride and sense of feeling self-sufficient.

Now, at sixty, with a third fusion and permanent pain and damage that will likely keep me from ever being pain-free, I've sadly become the master at letting go, working the grief cycle like a pro. Still, too often I find myself stuck in anger or depression, trying hard to not get stuck in these toxic feelings and be thankful for what I can still do. All my pain-free friends say, "It could be worse," and yes, it could. But with chronic pain many times it is difficult to see the silver lining: that I can still walk (a short ways with a brace and cane), that I got on Social Security Disability Insurance[4] (but can't live on the amount), that I need to find the joy in life (hard when I'm always grinding my teeth in pain).

Recently I found myself trying to help a new friend, plagued by serious migraines and related problems, come to terms with the loss of her health, ability to work, effect on her relationships, and so on. She had learned of the grief cycle when her husband died five years ago, but thought it was only for death. I've found this simple template useful through the years in my therapeutic work, showing parents and kids how to grieve the loss of their house, job, relationship, innocence, and so on.

I'd like to say I've used the grief cycle as much as I'll have to with my joint problems, but I know that is not true. Deterioration is deterioration, and thus there is an inevitable further decline in my future. Can I live another twenty or twenty-five years with increasing pain? I don't ponder that much (denial?) as there's little I can do about it until it happens. In the meantime, I'll keep doing what I still can, and trying to gracefully let go of what I can't.

---

4 Social Security Disability Insurance is a government benefit in the United States that some with disabilities are eligible to apply for.

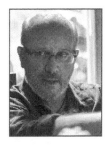

Before back and neck problems forced Bret onto disability benefits, he specialized in high-risk teenagers for almost thirty years, particularly gang youth. Three back and neck fusions unfortunately pulled him out of that work, but he keeps a few projects going through the pain. Bret is the author of From Boys to Men: Spiritual Rites of Passage in an Indulgent Age *and* The Undercurrents of Adolescence: Tracking the Evolution of Modern Adolescence and Delinquency Through Classic Cinema. *After twenty-six years in Lake Tahoe, Nevada, Bret is back in his hometown of Reno, Nevada, to get out of the snow!*

The Superior Mutant's Victory Garden

RAVEN KALDERA

Hubbardston, Massachusetts, United States

I'VE HAD LUPUS—SYSTEMIC lupus erythematosus—since puberty, but I didn't have a diagnosis until I was in my forties. That's not unusual for lupus—it can masquerade as so many different disorders that it often goes undiagnosed until it finally hits on the classic symptoms, which are rheumatoid arthritis and skin problems. I didn't connect the dots between the colitis; the chronic fatigue; the muscle pain; the allergies; the multiple chemical sensitivities; the freezing hands and feet; and the mysterious attacks of pneumonia, pleurisy, and liver dysfunction with no bacteria or viruses in evidence until the rheumatoid arthritis kicked in with a vengeance later in life. I come by my lupus genetically, and its initial onset was triggered by medication given to me around puberty for a genetic disorder of the adrenal glands that I also have. In addition, I have a mild to moderate case of Tourette syndrome, a seizure disorder, spatial dyslexia, a hiatal hernia, various internal organ deformations, and minor skeletal deformations of my spine and all my lower joints. In other words, I'm a deformed mutant! It's a pity that I didn't also inherit the ability to fly or turn into steel or bore holes through walls with my red-laser eyes, like the mutants in comic books.

I did, however, make the mutant connection early in life. I latched onto Marvel Comics' *Uncanny X-Men* instead of other comics, fantasizing about a world in which, even if your mismatched genes messed you up, they might also give you special gifts. Like many of the "mutants in hiding," I spent a lot of my resources hiding my disabilities. I'd choose clothing that camouflaged my body, make up excuses as to why I had to sit out gym class sometimes (the teachers knew, but the other kids would ask), and decorate my orthopedic shoes. I eventually decided to fix the inward pronation of my feet myself through an act of sheer willpower. I deliberately walked on the outer edges of my feet for a whole year whenever I was out of sight and managed to train them into something more normal-functioning. It was painful and awful, but it was one of my childhood triumphs.

This became my norm for dealing with chronic illness. I told myself that I was a tough motherfucker, and I hid pain and pushed through fatigue as best I could. I learned about herbs, diets, and other alternative medicine practices, and added them to my discipline. My mother had also suffered from chronic illnesses from the same genetic family, long before most of them were understood, so they weren't even diagnosable, much less treatable. She had resorted to vitamins and trace minerals and herbs to attempt to help her miserable existence. I asked her once about her pills, "Mama, if you're taking all of these, why are you still so sick all the time?" Her answer was, "You should see how bad I'd be if I wasn't taking all of these."

As I grew, my list of diagnoses got longer and longer along with physical difficulties; my fear was to end up like my mother, who spent whole days in bed and still other days half out of her head with mental illness, some of that caused by her physical illnesses. These days, while the lupus does land me in bed for days at a time, I consider myself lucky. Even with my mutant laundry list, I am very, very fortunate, because I did not inherit any of the specific problems that affected her ability to interact with reality. I have an able-bodied partner who suffers from a neu-rochemical mood disorder, so I know that when it's at its worst, he's just as disabled as I am. My mother bore both of those bur-dens, and it isn't surprising that she went down under them and was never able to get up again.

Of course, chronic pain—these days mostly from the rheu-matoid arthritis and the muscle tissue attacks—can create its own problems with cognitive thought. I call this the "Screaming Face" syndrome, and this is how I explain chronic pain to peo-ple who don't have it. Imagine that you wake up in the morning and there's a disembodied face hanging right in front of yours, blocking most of your field of vision. The face is screaming, not even in words, "Aaah! Aaah! Aaaaah!" All the time, nonstop. You will be using up a lot of your resources to block out the Scream-ing Face enough to get up, shower, dress, find some food, not to mention any work you might want to do. You have to speak over the Screaming Face, and your train of thought is often derailed. When I warn my partners that it's a Screaming Face day, they know that they will have to repeat statements, and that I may seem distanced or distracted, and it's not personal.

When I promised myself that I would not become my moth-er, my best tool was my willpower. If there was a problem, I'd tough it out, I'd push through it. If there were adaptations to make, I'd make them. If there was something that needed disci-pline to accomplish, like taking supplements or making dietary changes, I'd do it. Learn to meditate and breathe out the pain? Okay. Learn breathing techniques to break a lupus fever? Got it. Scrupulously study labels to avoid allergens and chemicals in food, even when that means not eating out? Can do. Wear that respirator when walking past a cloud of smokers, as it can land me in bed for a week? Fine. Face down each new and creative way that the Lupus Wolf finds to chew on my body with a goal-oriented plan of research and attack? Let me at it. Drag myself back from the edge of lupus-induced liver failure with herbs and supplements? Done. Make more dietary changes to cope with the new liver-induced diabetes? On it. I awe my primary care physician with my proactive approach, my attempts to dominate the Lupus Wolf, to be the alpha of the pack in this body by any means necessary.

The hardest parts, though, are when willpower doesn't work. With lupus, sometimes pushing through the pain instead of just giving up and going to bed for a couple of days will make the end result worse. Sometimes that means I'll eventually be in bed for a week anyway, when a couple of days' rest could have ended the flare sooner. This is a terrible disease for someone who is, as one of my partners calls me, a "Type A-plus." The gambling game of allocating one's spoons:[5] how many do I think I'll have today? Can I push through, or do I need to give up and fall over? What will pushing through do to me tomorrow? Can I skip this precaution, or will it endanger me? Will the treatment for this problem make this other problem worse? Can I get help for this thing I can no longer do myself? These considerations exhaust me, and they must be done every day no matter how badly I feel. There are moments when I just break down and weep, because it all seems so pointless and grim at that moment, in the grip of pain and fatigue and fever.

There is also the humiliation of a progressive and incurable disease; I watch myself be able to do less and less every year and have to ask for help with more and more activities. I can't buckle my own boots on any more, nor can I carry anything heavy. Sometimes I've had to be held up against the bathroom wall and washed down, because I couldn't do it myself. My wife is a very active and sporty person, and I can no longer accompany her on most of the outdoor activities we used to do together. Each time

---

5 Spoon Theory is a concept developed by Christine Miserandino and fully explained on her website at butyoudontlooksick.com. "Spoons" is often used as shorthand for the available capacity to manage fatigue and other symptoms of chronic illness.

I have to give up some piece of independence or ability, it's like a slap in the face. Each time I am reminded of it, for at least the first fifty times, will be another slap.

We've had to change the house. We now have an accessible tub where I can sit down, and we are putting in a new bedroom with a ramp to it, and a fully chair-accessible bathroom. I don't need those most of the time yet, but I'm pretty sure I will need them eventually. These changes came about because a friend with cerebral palsy was visiting. He's a disability activist, and he inquired about my health, and then asked me, "So when are you making the house accessible?" Making the effort now is being kind to future me, who will be cursing his own lack of accessibility. It's also being realistic about my limitations, which is always difficult for me to face. It's hard to be realistic about them while holding on to a hopeful, can-do attitude. It's hard, when your life is one step forward and two steps back, to be grateful about the one step forward.

It's very easy for me to fall into hating my body, and it's a very unhealthy place for me to live in. I dissociate quickly, and have a hard time feeling anything but resentful about my difficult flesh. I combat this through collecting positive sensations—nice fabrics, tasty food (given what I'm allowed on my limited diet), beautiful sights and smells, good massages, and great sex with my partners whenever I've got the time and spoons. I remind myself that I am still attractive to them, regardless of what the rest of the world thinks. I don't let myself be a "stereotypical crip." I put spikes and studs on my black plastic leg braces, I had my fierce-looking motocross boots altered to be ankle braces, and I'm going to decorate my boss red wheelchair with barbaric furs and sheepskins. I try to find a daily discipline of looking for joy in small things, and especially small good things my body can experience. I tell myself again and again that it's worth being here in a body that can feel, even if much of what it feels isn't pleasant.

Pain comes and goes for me. Some days it's mild, some days belong to the Screaming Face. Occasional days are even pain-free, and other occasional days are spent in bed, rocking back and forth. The pain issue is made worse by the fact that nearly all painkillers are off-limits to me. Because my immune system is crazed, I can become allergic to anything at any time. At some point I became allergic to ibuprofen because I was taking it daily. The doctors warned me that allergies to nonsteroidal anti-inflammatories (NSAIDs) tend to spread through that entire family of drugs over time, and indeed that's just what happened.

I was taking so many NSAIDs because I am pretty much entirely resistant to opioid-based drugs, which is an anecdotal side effect of Tourette syndrome. I know several fellow Touretters with chronic pain who have the same awful problem. I discovered this when I came out of surgery for the first time and found out—while lying there with 108 stitches—that no opioid-based painkiller up to and including morphine would do anything but make me sleepy. The pain never stopped. Those four days post-surgery were one of the worst ordeals of my life, second only to my near-death experience from bleeding out due to a perfect storm of endocrinal and internal organ malfunction. What do I do? I get a lot of acupuncture, both professionally and at home. I get massage and acupressure, and I do a lot of meditating and breathing out the pain. And I hold out hope that my doctors will eventually be able to come up with a new painkiller that works for me, as medical science advances.

I've also faced down death. It's entirely likely that my bodily malfunctions will kill me someday; unless I'm hit by a bus or something, complications from lupus are the most likely candidate for my death. By the time it was discovered, I was already allergic to corticosteroids, which is the front-line treatment for autoimmune diseases. People with non-medicable lupus tend not to live that long. I've come within shouting distance of the door of death on a couple of occasions now, and I've outlived several doctors' predictions for me. I'm closing in on fifty and I'm still above ground. Pain, while usually my enemy, also reminds me that I'm still alive. I tell myself this over and over, while I'm breathing it out, while I'm distracting myself with some good and beautiful thing in my life. I'm still alive, and I'm still able to enjoy this. Be grateful. For the moment, it's enough. I am the Superior Mutant, and despite all its efforts, my DNA hasn't killed me yet.

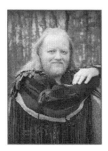

Raven Kaldera is a Superior Mutant living on a little homestead farm in Massachusetts with his polyamorous family, most of whom are also Superior Mutants in various ways. He is a shaman, a spiritual teacher, the author of thirty-nine books, and he struggles every day to be a better person.

Growing Up with Asthma

MARK LUDAS

West Orange, New Jersey, United States

LIVING WITH CHRONIC ASTHMA as an adult is somewhat easier than being an asthmatic child. Nowadays, I am so familiar with the feelings, the stresses, the urgencies of being unable to breathe, that sometimes when I'm working out at the gym and pushing myself I wonder if I've become too blasé about my condition. Maybe I push myself too hard sometimes, convinced that as long as I have my inhaler in my pocket, nothing bad will happen. It's like I have something to prove. Will there come a day when my pride and my defiance get me into trouble? When the wheezing becomes so bad that I can't get enough oxygen to my brain and I fall over? Pass out? Gym floors are usually only padded in a few places.

It's incredible to think that I can be so easygoing about not being able to breathe. As a child, my attitude was not so "whatever." Panic comes more easily when you haven't survived these symptoms a million times over.

One public service announcement I heard describes the feeling of asthmatic symptoms as "[being] like a fish with no water." I like to say it's more like running into a burning building. Maybe I attach the sensation of running to it because I have exercise-induced asthma. Whenever I tried to join the other boys playing in the yard, running around and laughing, my window of enjoyment was very small. My laugh became a cough, whereas theirs didn't. I inevitably had to sit down and use the inhaler or nebulizer.

The same is true today. Despite any successes at the gym, that moment always comes when I have to say, "Okay, I need to stop for a moment." And I'll usually use my inhaler. Thankfully, I probably won't need the nebulizer again until I'm a senior citizen. I still have one though, just in case.

As a child I received a book called *Don't You Dare Shoot That Bear* for my birthday one year. It was about Theodore Roosevelt and his experiences as the archetypal "grab life by the horns" kind of person. I read about him extensively, and learned that he overcame his childhood asthma through athletic activity, like boxing. So I asked for and received a punching bag for my tenth birthday.

I was eleven when I tried to muster Roosevelt's resolve. The Presidential Fitness Test was in full effect at school, and it involved running a mile. All my life, in gym class I'd been allowed to sit out whenever I wanted. For the mile run, I was given the option of walking it. But I had a special, unique feeling that year. I didn't want to be last in my class. I decided I would run it the whole way.

And when I crossed the finish line, in first place, I fell to the ground, unable to breathe. My friend Shawn walked me to the nurse, where I spent the rest of the day. I was elated. I had had a taste of being athletic, of being physically exceptional. I guess that young boy mirrors who I am today, with something to prove to himself, who would say, "Screw it, I'm going to run," instead of being content to remain defined by his health condition.

I sometimes consider that maybe Roosevelt's overcoming asthma is just part of his myth. On the other hand, from what I understand, there are children who do outgrow their asthma. I never did. Sometimes it irritates me, and sometimes I don't mind at all. It would be nice to feel safe being active, to feel robust and with fewer limits on my physical expression. At the same time though, my asthma has helped make me the compassionate, thoughtful person I am.

Now, as a certified personal trainer, I know all too well the various levels of fright and doubt that can arise in a person's mind at the adverse feelings induced by exercise. I certainly know what it's like to associate exercise with discomfort, which for me was a physical sensation not unlike drowning, inhaling smoke, or having a fifty-pound weight on your chest. As a result, I know how to articulate the feelings of pain that are often necessary to produce "gain."

Unlike a lot of other trainers who were born athletic, I possess the compassion and patience that are required when trying to help someone prove to themselves that they can change their own life. And I'm grateful for that compassion, for that patience. Most importantly perhaps, I'm able to help people work with their physical limitations, not deny them or shame them. If they can accept these things as part of who they are as I did, they can at least start to overcome the psychological implications of being different, if not also the physical.

In this way, I have overcome my asthma. Even though I sometimes end up gasping on the treadmill, or taking minutes to catch my breath between heavy squats. Running another mile like I did in fifth grade seems like a bit of stretch (though at least I know I could do it, and will again), but it doesn't shape who I am. It is only one part of me, just like my inhaler is only one thing I carry.

In addition to that, having asthma has produced one other positive outcome: it has helped me decide which athletic shorts to buy. No pockets, no deal.

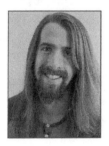

Mark Ludas is a published author, accomplished actor and musician, and blogger on a wide range of subject matter. He is also a private personal trainer in northern New Jersey and a lifelong copyeditor, currently working in that capacity for Jerrick Media Holdings, Inc., in Englewood, New Jersey.

Part 5

Things We Wish We'd Known

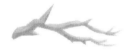

Things Every Newly Diagnosed Patient Needs to Know

DYLAN GOMEZ

San Jose, California, United States

WHEN I WAS FIRST diagnosed in 2011 with Crohn's disease, a chronic illness, I didn't know what "chronic," "incurable disease," or even "diagnosis" meant. It's not that I didn't understand the definitions; I didn't know what they meant for me. I've experienced symptoms related to my Crohn's since I was two years old, though I grew up not knowing why. I had inexplicable pain, I couldn't eat, and I didn't understand why I had to have blood drawn when other kids didn't. And there were never any answers.

When I finally got my diagnosis, the doctors gave me the impression that since they determined the problem, fixing it would be an easy matter. They didn't explain the severity or progression of my disease to me. They didn't tell me about the lifestyle changes I'd need to make. They made it sound like managing my disease and achieving remission were the same as a cure. There are many things I wish I could travel back in time to tell myself. But I can't change my past. Instead, I can do my best to help the future of those who are now where I was.

1. Your pain is real, and valid. There will be times when your doctors won't know what is causing your pain, or why nothing relieves it. They may seem to blame it on you. They will forget that you are suffering, and start to doubt you instead of doubting their own abilities. Don't ever let anyone tell you that your pain isn't real or is all in your head. You don't have to prove your pain to anyone for it to be real.

2. You can say no. Activities, procedures, taking medications, answering questions; you do not have to engage in anything you don't want to. You can reject invasive exams and procedures you are uncomfortable with. You are not obligated to lie about how you feel or say yes for the sake of others. Feel free to just say no.

3. You will not have one final better moment. You will have many better moments. People who do not have or know someone with a chronic illness tend to think there is a final remedy for everything, that once you start feeling better, you won't be sick again. What they don't understand is that chronic illness comes with ups and downs. We have good days and bad days. We don't know how we are going to feel in three minutes, three hours, or three weeks. What we do know is there will always be better moments and days to come.

4. You don't need to entertain every suggestion. "Have you tried thinking positively? Eating healthy? Exercise? Praying? An obscure cure from the internet?" Though these suggestions come with good intentions, you can ignore them or even ask that they stop trying to find easy solutions to a complex problem.

5. You don't have to be productive or cured to be worthy, inspiring, or amazing. If you want to comfort and help others, do it. Even just running a blog or talking to someone

on the phone can make a difference. You don't have to get better to follow a dream. Do whatever your heart tells you, and don't be discouraged by your health.

6. You don't have to inspire other people, set an example, or find a lesson in this. If you don't want to inspire other people or be a public example, you don't have to. You can be whoever the heck you want to be. Your illness is yours and does not need to be framed as a fulfilling journey or life lesson just because others want to see that Hollywood spin. You have gone through a lot, and you don't have to fit a cookie-cutter version of chronic illness to validate that. Don't feel obligated to sugarcoat your life to fabricate an inspirational story; illnesses are not pretty or fun, and you do not need to hide this.

7. Not all doctors are respectful or noble people. If you are not getting the care or respect you need, switch. You will meet invalidating, compassionless, and disrespectful doctors, but you will also meet some incredibly caring doctors. Treatments, procedures, and health decisions are a lot easier when you have a doctor who understands and respects you. So don't be afraid to search until you find the right one.

8. This illness is not a punishment for any reason. People will always try to put a positive spin on your situation for their own comfort. Some may say this is punishment from the universe or from God without considering how that makes you feel. You are not responsible for your illness. You haven't done anything wrong. Sometimes things just happen without a reason.

9. Planning your schedule around your illness does not mean you are letting your illness define you. Illnesses are unpredictable, inconsiderate, and can be ruthless. This means planning events can be equally unpredictable. You will

have times where you don't have a choice. Your illness doesn't define you because you are working around it. Don't feel like you've failed or given up if you're forced to move appointments or miss an event.

10. **You are trying hard enough.** Don't let anyone, whether they have a chronic illness or not, judge how hard you're trying. You are trying hard enough; even when you aren't trying. These people will never understand this concept or how their comments affect us. Don't let them get in your head, or feel the need to listen.

11. **Everyone's illness is different.** Don't let anyone invalidate you because your disease isn't cancer, or because someone they know with this illness has gotten better. Illnesses can't and shouldn't be compared. Many people, both ill and not ill, will play "who has it worse." There's no reason to compete for the title of Most Ill Person In All Existence. When it comes to illnesses, complications, symptoms, medications, etc., everyone is different and it isn't a game.

12. **You are a human being, not just a patient or an illness.** Doctors can forget that your mental health takes a toll in all of this. They order treatments and procedures without asking how we are doing emotionally. Many of them don't even realize that invalidating our concerns makes us doubt ourselves even more. Don't feel bad if you need to stop a session. When you are right in between the scale of feeling bad and good, but you feel stuck since you aren't improving at all and feel unheard—that's Chronic Illness Limbo. If you feel your quality of life is being overlooked, it's okay to speak up.

13. **Your priorities may change after you get sick.** Your big goals may have to turn into smaller goals, and that's okay. Don't feel bad if your previous goals for higher education or travel turn into a single goal to just get out of bed in the

morning. Goals and priorities will change as your situation changes, so don't feel like you've failed if previous goals are replaced by smaller ones. Taking care of yourself is your biggest priority, and you're achieving great things by focusing on that.

14. Don't let anyone dictate how you're supposed to feel or what outlook you're supposed to have. It's okay to feel down or defeated, and it's okay to stand tall and feel strong. It's okay to feel invincible, and it's okay to feel like you're tired of it all. It's okay to accept your situation or still be in denial. Whatever you may feel, whether it's positive or not, is valid. Even the negative feelings. Do your best not to become consumed by them, but regardless, you're not alone.

15. Use non-harmful coping mechanisms that work for you. Whether it's having a Netflix marathon, singing at the top of your lungs, creating art, writing stories, meditating, reading, or something else, you will find something that helps you cope. If people tell you that doing something else is better than what you're already doing, don't feel obligated to listen. Do what you feel is best for you, because you are the one who is going through this battle. You know you best.

16. People who are not sick will never understand your struggle as much as you want them to. The people who love you will try their best to understand. Even if they don't fully understand, they will still be there to comfort you and fight with you. If you lose friends because they did not understand or try to, it means that they weren't worth your time in the first place. As much as we try to educate people, we can't force compassion. You are not and should never feel like a burden. You can cut ties with anyone at any time; don't feel in debt to someone because they were there for you in the past or because you used to be close

friends. Your genuine friends will stick around and be there for you, and they are the ones worth your time.

17. You are not obligated to talk about it in detail if you don't want to. Family members and friends will occasionally step over your comfortable boundaries and ask about your illness. They may feel like it's their chance to play doctor and tell you how you should fix yourself. In situations like these, don't feel obligated to talk about it or listen to their suggestions. This is your body, not theirs. Physical illnesses are as personal as a divorce, and many people forget that. If a couple was in the process of divorcing, it would not be acceptable to go up to them and ask things like: "Have you tried doing _____ to fix it?" "How's your divorce going?" "Maybe your marriage fell apart because _____." "I know a guy who had that same kind of divorce but he did _____ and it was magically fixed!" So why would it be acceptable to ask those things about a chronic illness? It's not.

18. Don't be afraid to ask for help or feel guilty if you need to ask a favor from someone. Whether it's because you need a ride to an appointment, help cleaning your house, someone to help you study, or someone to run errands with, it's always okay to ask for help. The people who truly love and support you will always be there in your time of need in whatever capacity they can be. If someone gives you permission to contact them immediately when you need help, don't hesitate to take them up on that offer. Even the strongest people need help sometimes.

There are other situations and reassurances I could add, but those are the things you'll learn best by experiencing them yourself. Don't feel obligated to follow what I've said; always do what you decide is best for you and puts you first.

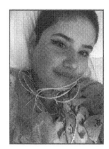

Dylan Gomez is a chronically ill nineteen-year-old who wrote this piece while in a hospital bed for many months. In their free time, they enjoy filmmaking, reading comic books, volunteering and fundraising for the Crohn's and Colitis Foundation of America, and writing relatable (and sometimes humorous) content on their personal blog to help people who are also suffering from chronic illnesses feel understood and to give them a laugh. Dylan hopes to soon complete a film with Baykids Studios that will talk about what it's like to live with inflammatory bowel disease.

Wishing I Had a Heads-Up on My Autoimmune Illnesses

JAMIE JASINSKI

Westville, New Jersey, United States

I DO NOT BELIEVE that everything happens for a reason, or that there is a master plan laid out for me to blindly follow. I think those are things that people fall back on when they don't know what else to say in bad circumstances. What I do believe in is trying to find something positive even in the worst situations. I've lived the past year and a half silently suffering from chronic illness, and only my closest friends and family members know the truth. I've been embarrassed of myself and what my life has become during this trying time. However, I recently found that writing about my struggles, even if only for the two people who follow my blog, has been my glass half full. I want others to realize and understand what it is that we, as a community with chronic and invisible illnesses, face daily.

My life has never been as sad, repetitive, and anxiety-ridden as it is now. If there's one thing that I wish, it's for me to have known that something like this was coming so I could have done a lot more of what I loved beforehand: running along the beach, theme park excursions, hours of shopping—all things that I cannot do anymore but reflect back on. I wish I had known that I needed to slow down in my daily life and really take care of myself, both mentally and physically, before my diagnosis came. We cannot go back though, so all I have is the motion of going forward and trying to find inner peace and some sense of happiness.

There's no book or conversation that can prepare you for how you are going to cope with your illness. There are online resources that can help you in knowing others are going through similar struggles, but we are all different, and we all deal with and react to our circumstances in our own way. I have a family history of autoimmune disease, but I never expected it to come my way. It came fast, and it attacked my body in ways that I wasn't prepared for. I have rheumatoid arthritis and Sjögren's syndrome, both of which destroy your healthy tissues. As I mentioned, it is over a year, and I'm still trying to find medications that work for me. I'm not even anywhere close to a point where I can take a deep breath and relax.

My biggest struggle with my chronic illnesses has been those in my world who cannot grasp that I am sick because I suffer from invisible illnesses. I am sick. Hang around in my apartment for a few hours, and you will witness it firsthand. It's at these times that I want to get angry, but can I blame them? I was just as naive about my diseases upon being diagnosed until I properly educated myself.

In fact, the doctor who diagnosed me never even explained that I would have these things for the rest of my life. It wasn't until I went to my primary care doctor that the severity of what I was dealing with was explained to me; that day, I had a huge reality check. My thinking was no longer short-term, but long, and it was no longer how to reduce my symptoms quickly, but to find a way to live with them comfortably. I'm learning to listen to my body, resting when I feel the slightest bit of tiredness, not forcing myself to keep trucking along because I don't want others to perceive me a certain way. I'm learning to share my feelings more, so people can understand what I am going through, rather than shutting down and internalizing it all. I'm learning to advocate for myself, something that is so very scary and new to me. Most importantly, I'm learning that I am strong. I've wanted to give up many times, but I've managed to find a way to tell myself that I need to keep going. There must be a way to find my happy place again, and I am eager to find it.

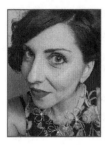 *Jamie Jasinski is from New Jersey and loves every minute of being a dog mom to her rescue pup that supports her emotionally. She has been diagnosed with rheumatoid arthritis, Sjögren's syndrome, and fibromyalgia. She writes about her experiences with these autoimmune diseases and advocates for those living with chronic illness. You can follow her on her personal journey by visiting her pieces at themighty.com/u/jamie-jasinski.*

Along the Way

DESS

Savannah, Georgia, United States

OVER THE PAST TWO years, I've been diagnosed with endometriosis, hidradenitis suppurativa, interstitial cystitis, and irritable bowel syndrome. I never thought my life would change so drastically in my twenties! At times, it's been difficult navigating through the world of chronic illness. Before this I was a regular college student. I did my best to pass my classes, work, hang out with friends, and get involved in campus activities. But somewhere along the way, I started getting sick. I'd ignored some symptoms I'd had since high school (occasional headaches, fatigue, nausea, constipation, pelvic pain, etc.) But they lingered and got worse; I couldn't ignore them anymore. Simple things like getting up to attend class became a challenge. I went to the health center at my university for advice. They couldn't do much, so my parents recommended seeing a doctor in town to find out what was going on. That marked the beginning of my journey. Here are a few things I've learned along the way:

Setting up Doctor's Appointments on My Own

Before getting diagnosed with chronic illnesses, my parents always set up doctor's visits for me. I didn't need to do it myself until I had to see doctors all the time. I was terrified I'd embarrass myself or say something stupid when making an appointment. But it wasn't so bad. After a few calls, it got easier.

Finding Doctors

In the beginning, I wasn't sure where to find a doctor. I couldn't see my pediatrician anymore because I was too old. Where was I supposed to go? What kind of doctors did adults see? I didn't know, so I went to a doctor my family recommended. In the beginning it was great. I was finally going to a doctor for grown-ups. But it didn't work out, so I found another doctor who's been amazing. They helped me figure out what to do next. They explained that people see primary care physicians (PCPs) once they're eighteen or older, and PCPs refer people to specialists that treat specific conditions. I'm thankful they shared that info with me. Now, I see a PCP and specialists for my chronic illnesses.

Getting Insurance

Before I was sick, I didn't think I needed insurance. I wised up after I had to pay for appointments, surgeries, medications, and more by myself. The medical bills burned a hole in my pocket. A huge chunk of my paychecks from work were used to chip away at previous medical bills I couldn't pay at the time. I felt stuck. After seeing me struggle, family and friends advised me get health insurance. Once I did, I could finally breathe again. It didn't make my old medical bills disappear, but it helped reduce costs by a lot. If you see multiple doctors, make sure your insurance plan includes all of them. If not, it may cause problems down the road. I learned that the hard way.

Getting Around a Hospital/Health Center

When I began seeing my doctors, I'd get lost trying to find their offices. I was super nervous about seeing them, so I was a mess. I learned a few things to make it easier; Google Maps became my best friend. The days of getting lost were over. And getting to the hospital/health center early made a difference. How would I know where to go once I got inside the building?

I couldn't use my GPS for that. I would look for a map or ask someone at the front desk for directions. That's seems obvious, right? Yeah, but it took me a while to figure a lot out. I was anxious and hated asking for help.

Speaking Up at the Doctor's Office

Advocating for myself was never a skill I excelled in. As a kid, I depended on family and friends to speak up for me. I had to speak up for myself at the doctor's office though. At my initial appointments, I received lots of information. Most of it went over my head and I wasn't sure how to handle it. I wondered if it was better to ask questions or stay silent. But there were questions in my mind I couldn't ignore. What do all these words I'm hearing mean? Will my illnesses get worse? Will these medications really help? Do I have to change my diet? Do I need surgery? How are these illnesses going to affect my life? Do I have a say in how to deal with this? Although I was scared, I shared my thoughts with each doctor. They answered my questions and took my concerns into consideration then, and still do now. It took a long time to find doctors like that, but I'm glad I found them. If a doctor ignores your concerns or doesn't treat you well, find another one who will. Everyone deserves to be treated with respect.

To anyone reading this, you are not alone. Living with a chronic illness can be isolating sometimes. But there are resources online to connect and get advice from others who know what you're going through. Hang in there; you're amazing.

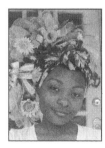

Dess lives in Savannah, Georgia. She loves to read, try new recipes, and watch Netflix.

I Wish I'd Known

ZOE A. BATEMAN

Reading, United Kingdom

THE LITTLE GIRL FELL over in the playground, ankle twisted around. The girl watched as others screamed and ran for help. Her teacher turned white. I wish she'd known it wasn't normal. I wish she'd known that ankles shouldn't be able to be pulled back together by tiny hands and that pain wasn't normal. I wish she'd known she didn't have to put up a brave face. I wish she'd known that it was okay to cry, that she wasn't weak. I wish she had known that she was braver than all the other kids. I wish she had known that she was amazing for walking on that ankle as it crunched beneath her. Her family didn't realize it was dislocated when it went back so easily. I wish she had known.

The young girl wonders about fire and brimstone, because how much worse can it be than the life she is already living? Only twelve years old, but she knows something isn't right. The girl who writes with pain streaking along her arm, who cannot put down the words she means to because she can't handle the pain anymore. I wish she had known it was the teachers failing her, not the other way around. They should have known something was wrong when she spoke so well and wrote so badly. Her handwriting should have shown them the storm inside her mind. I wish she could have known how she'd prove them wrong. I wish she wasn't called lazy. I wish she had known that she put in more effort than anyone. I wish she could have known how proud everyone would be when they realized what she accomplished while fighting the agony. I wish she had known that the princesses in the books she read to escape would have looked up to her. I know I do. I just wish she knew.

The teen girl whose veins are alight with pain pushes herself further than most, trying not to be a wimp. The girl did a marathon at fourteen, walked all the way, cried the last six miles, but did it. She was the youngest that year. The girl couldn't stand or move for days afterward, crying in pain, not understanding why others healed so quickly. I wish someone had told her she didn't have to try so hard. I wish someone told her she wasn't lesser than them. I wish someone had sat her down and told her destroying herself was not the answer.

I wish someone had held the breaking girl, telling her the pain did not make her weak. I wish she had known what a feat she had accomplished. I wish she hadn't felt the need to do it, but I am proud that she did. I wish she hadn't felt that despair, and I wish she had known that what she was doing was destroying her. I wish she had known she wasn't a failure. I wish she had known doctors would look at her with amazement in their eyes. I wish she knew that this wasn't the answer.

The young adult buys her first cane. She is unable to walk, and barely able to stand. When it arrives, what little confidence she had built before is burned to the ground. There are advertisements on the packaging, all with photos of people seventy years or older. The ads are not for her. The girl who breaks down and is unable to get back up. The girl who finally found some freedom only to see it slammed in her face. I wish she had known that breaking down was okay. I wish she had known that the cane would help. I wish she had known that her diagnosis did not make her old.

The girl sits in the same bed as me. She can barely sit up due to pain but smiles at everyone. The girl holds back her screams as her body burns with pain. She can barely move, but can finally stand up for herself. The girl can't shower; she hates herself for being everything femininity is not. I wish she had known how strong she was. I wish she had known her tears were a sign of how strong she tried to be for so long. I wish she had known that being her is enough. I wish she had known that being strong is overrated.

I tell these things to the girls who I once was. I wish I had known that the teachers were wrong. I wish I had known that they had failed me. I wish I had known that the pain in my veins was not universal, that my life was deemed harder by genetics chosen before I was born. That I was valid.

I wish I could believe all of this. I believe it for them. For the six-year-old girl who learned to walk on feet of coal. For the twelve-year-old girl who could not make sense of the pain that others seemed to overcome. For the eighteen-year-old girl who was finally breaking. I believe it for them. For the girls I used to be. So why not for me? The girl lying in the bed? The one who defies doctors by continuing her degree, the girl who gets sicker as time goes on. She is strong too. I just wish I knew that sooner.

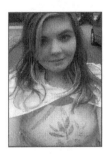

Zoe A. Bateman is a British author. She is usually found trying to hug her cats or finding creative ways to do physio exercises.

If I Had Known Then, What I Know Now...

MARCIA ALLAR

Newton, Massachusetts, United States

MOST OF MY THOUGHTS following that sentence—if I had known then, what I know now—seem trite, or like a "perverted positive" lesson learned from a terrible incident. But I often think about how, in two, three, or five years from now, I don't want to be thinking, "If I had known then what I know now," with the "then" referring to today. This makes me wonder how I could take the lessons learned from before and send them into the future to avoid regrets. This emphasizes the importance of being in the now right now, and living an improved, cleaner, simpler, and calmer life.

A mental handbook of what I have learned seems to be falling off the tips of my fingers onto the computer keys:

1. I would have worried less, because now I know that most of what I worry about never happens and the things that happen I never even worried about.

2. I would have relaxed more and been more present with my children, friends, and myself. I try to slow myself down now and this lets me notice more nature, the sounds of my friends' voices, thoughts of what my dog is looking at from

her little point of view. This helps me to be more present in life, rather than just moving through it.

3. I would have trusted my intuition more. It is so clear to me now how I can sense what is and is not right, and how listening to that inner me then directs my actions. It is a perverse positive, because by not listening before, I was injured by doctors, situations, and people. It led to present illnesses, causing me to be homebound and in constant pain. Now I really try to listen to what I am feeling about a situation. I try to give more space and room for that type of dialogue in my head, which is otherwise overfilled with senseless worry or old, patterned dialogues. It is so important to feel a sense of myself, and more importantly to avoid questioning whether the right people are helping or harming me.

4. I would have stopped trying to fix and change people so much. As a nurse, and then as a lawyer for injured people, I could play out my "I can fix it" desires that came from wishing someone had "fixed it" for me. Now I realize that I can assist or offer advice that may or may not be taken and try hard to not be attached to the outcome.

5. I would have made room for more fun. I love to watch television now as a break, but I used to think that it was a waste of time and silly. It's good to be silly, and why rush the other things I have to get done? They are never-ending. Like an endless rope of beads with nothing at the end to keep them from falling off. Whether it was taking care of my family, my children, or my friends, taking care of myself was always at the end of the beads. The priorities were off.

6. I would have taken the time to grieve my losses and feel my sadness. I have found that they all come back years, sometimes decades later and hit me on the head with the strength of a ton of bricks. Being mad protected me from

feeling sad. Now I can feel "smad" (a combo) and try to tease out the sad and feel it. When my feelings are really felt, they can be heard and then can be released to wherever they go in this universe. My feelings are like little upset children, and once they feel like they are listened to, they can maybe calm down. I took a big sigh just writing that; to be relieved of them is wonderful and makes so much room for better, good things to come back into that space of my inner life.

7. I would have been more open to exploring new ways to heal. Now I have practitioners that lead me to different approaches with the hope of getting better. I fully understand now that the way the universe works is way beyond my understanding. Energy work done by a physician in New York can help me or be too much for me sometimes. That would have been unthinkable for me to consider or believe before. But now that I've experienced it, I believe it is real for sure. Being open to totally different ways to heal my body and soul has led to feeling better even if I can't understand it.

8. I would have given myself credit for being, "Braver than [I] believe[d] and stronger than [I] seem[ed] and smarter than [I] thought]."[6] I am mindful that I can be all those things and move forward with confidence instead of my inner demons of doubt and insecurity.

I made a list in 1983 when I was taking my first mindfulness course, when my chronic pain syndrome began. It has been sitting in my closet for thirty years with me occasionally glancing at it but never taking it in.

• Accept more

---

6 From the film *Pooh's Grand Adventure: The Search for Christopher Robin*, released in 1997. Directed by Karl Geurs; story by A. A. Milne.

- Trust more

- Nurture more

- Relax more

- Hope more

- Experience more

- Enjoy more

- Heal more

- Forgive more, and

- Remember the most difficult battle is the internal one

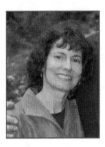

Marcia Allar lives with complex regional pain syndrome, chemical sensitivities, Ehlers-Danlos syndrome, and osteoporosis. She was an oncology head nurse and then a trial attorney for severely injured people in Boston, Massachusetts. She now provides environmental counseling regarding healthy homes, nontoxic products, clean water, and safe foods. She lives in Newton, Massachusetts with her beloved dog, Sophie, and is the mother of two adult children, Sarah and Ben.

Part 6

What We Wish Folks Knew

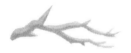

Chronically Ill Teens

MICHAELA SHELLEY

Spartanburg, South Carolina, United States

I THINK PEOPLE OFTEN forget about the sick teenagers. We aren't adults yet, but we aren't little kids either. We can understand what the doctors are doing to us and why. Sadly, what comes with that is knowing that sometimes we are going to have to feel worse before we can feel better. We are sick at a time in our lives where otherwise we feel invincible. We think nothing can ever stop us in this world and then, boom, life picks you out of nowhere and you are stuck in a position where you don't have a choice. Life isn't in your control anymore. As teenagers we want to have that control, and without that, it makes it hard to cope.

Teenagers can understand what's happening even if we don't fully get it. We don't have the experience adults have, which can make things confusing and complicated at times. All these emotions get mixed up in our heads and we become frustrated and angry. Even adults know it is hard keeping emotions in check. Being sick and dealing with the added emotions—on top of trying to manage normal teenager aspects of life—is quite the ordeal.

What if you needed someone to help you get up to go to the bathroom, to walk, to shower, to give you your needed medications, to take you to your doctor's appointments, and to be there at the hospital with you during your stays almost around the clock? I think that is difficult for a grown adult to grasp, much less a teenager. We are at an age where we are gaining more independence than we ever have before: going out with friends without your parents, driving, heading off to college, and building a life for yourself. Just imagine being fourteen or eighteen and suddenly having everything stripped from you. All your newfound independence is gone.

Our friends can't really relate to us anymore because they don't understand. They don't know what it's like to be sick and not have the energy to get out of bed in the morning. We want to go to school but we can't. Missing out on social events and the daily aspects of life for hospital stays, treatments, and doctor appointments makes us feel isolated. We don't want to lose our friends. Life goes on with or without you, and sadly, when you are sick, life often has to go on without you. You have that isolated feeling like no one understands you. There's no one to relate to, and you certainly aren't a normal teenager anymore. It is hard enough being a teenager and having to figure out what you want to make of yourself and grow up to be. Adding on a chronic illness makes that ten times harder.

Sometimes I feel like life hates me. I can never win this war and just because I want something to turn out one way doesn't always mean it is going to. Ninety-eight percent of the time, life doesn't go my way. If life went my way, then I wouldn't be sick. I wouldn't have all these diseases that people can't pronounce or have never heard of in their life. I wouldn't have all these tubes sticking out of my body, and I can certainly tell you I would not be taking all these pills that I'm taking now. I would be healthy, I'd be back to playing soccer, attending school every day, and I'd graduate on time.

It's expected that adults will get sick as they get older. Teenagers aren't supposed to be sick. We should be the healthy, high school star athletes, but not all of us can be. Some of us have grown up being sick and in the hospital, but to others it's a whole new world. Younger kids don't know what's happening. They are left in the dark about many things; they don't know if their treatment plan is even working. But teenagers know. We experience the bad news firsthand. We see our parents cry and we understand that pain. We cry too, because we know something bad and scary is happening. We've already been exposed to life as it is, and we know what is supposed to happen and what isn't.

Most importantly, we are not little kids, so don't treat us like that. We are not five; we are aware of and very capable of understanding what is going on in our bodies. We are just like any other young adult, except we have these extra challenges in front of us. Our disease does not inhibit our ability to comprehend what you are saying. For most of us, our brain is the exact same now as it was before our diagnosis a year or two ago.

All I am asking is that you don't forget us. Treat us like any other teen would be treated, just understand that we may not be able to do everything our peers can. Sometimes it might be hard for us to express how we feel when so many emotions overwhelm us. It can be hard for us to share with you exactly how we feel, because most days we don't even know. We are not adults and we are certainly not children. Our lives differ very much from them in how you need to treat the disease and how you need to treat us. It's certainly an unexpected journey and it is not an easy one either. All I ask is that you treat us like any normal teenager, be willing to help us along the way, and also give us some space. That's the only thing we truly want.

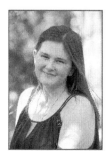

Michaela Shelley is a college student living with mitochondrial disease. She writes about her and her brother's experiences with the disease on her blog: chronicallyawesome23.blogspot.com.

All About the Pain

NIKKI ALBERT

Leduc, Alberta, Canada

I HAVE TWO CHRONIC pain conditions: fibromyalgia and chronic migraines. I say migraine and people say, "Ouch, that sounds like a bad headache." I say back, "I'll give you a bad headache," in a low, threatening tone. You see, while people fundamentally understand the concept of pain, they are not going to understand chronic pain unless they have felt a great deal of it for an extended period. It's a members-only club, I'm afraid. It is like understanding what a number is and then trying to understand what counting to infinity is like. Eventually it will just boggle your mind. Pain without an end boggles the mind.

Pain is a good thing. It is necessary. It is there to tell you there is some malfunction in the body that you really ought to pay attention to right now, preferably before you bleed to death or a predator catches you. That sort of fundamental function. Chronic pain is a malfunction; the system is broken. The signal won't shut down. There is no injury, there is just the pain signal on constant repeat. You just want to scream at your brain to shut the hell up already and that you get it. Or at the very least you wish there was a volume dial to turn down when the off button is broken.

How do you come to grips with a pain that has no cure and no end date? It is no easy task. It is, in fact, an impossible task.

People ask me how I cope with the pain all the time and I have no clue how to answer that question. I often just make crap up, so they don't realize how seriously close to not coping I am. The reality of chronic pain is a harsh one that even I don't like to look at too closely. One answer though, is that pain has time-warping abilities, with time and pain both being relative to the observer. Getting through the pain in the moment becomes the goal. Then getting through the day. The week. The next week. You lose your concept of the passage of time because your focus is getting through the moment. You must function somehow because that is what people expect, so you have to use every ounce of energy you have to do what is required of you.

So you survive pain, but you don't really get much else done. Also, you don't exactly remember much of anything. It is difficult to make long-term memories if you are in a boatload of pain. Things just slip through the gaps because your concentration really wasn't on what was happening. It was on the pain and only somewhat on what was happening. It makes for hazy memories and a distorted perception of the flow of time. Even your short-term memory and your feel for the passage of time is skewed by how much pain you are in. You lose a lot of time. That is less about coping and more about survival, but it is what it is. Occasionally, you reflect and realize how much time has passed and how much farther you have to go. Then you realize that is a painful realization. So you stop thinking about the future and the past.

Then, there is that amazing pain tolerance those of us with chronic pain have. It is our super power. Immense pain tolerance and the ability to grin and bear it. Some people think pain tolerance has something to do with willpower. Like they do a workout and it hurts a little, but they use their willpower and power through it. Victory is theirs. Wow. I'm impressed. They endured a little bit of pain for a very short duration. That's how I get out of bed in the morning.

Pain tolerance is something we learn as we go along. It is a behavior and that behavior is called "pretend you are not in pain so you can function in the real world." It's a facade you use to get through the day that becomes a reality. Pain tolerance is just a matter of being in pain, sometimes a great deal of pain, and not running around screaming or calling for an ambulance. Obviously, over time, moderate pain becomes a sort of baseline normal existence. That is pain tolerance. That amount of pain would cause someone without chronic pain to think there was something seriously wrong with their body. If you only ever had mild tension headaches once a decade and then one day got an acute migraine, you might think your head was about to implode.

There is a point where the facade breaks down, because your brain shuts down. You focus every bit of energy on trying to function and understand what people are saying and you have a sort of "zombie look." A glazed, empty look in the eye. A total lack of expression. The inability to really understand what people are saying and difficulty forming sentences. But if you ask me how I'm doing 99 percent of the time I'll say, "I'm fine," because that's how we roll. We get used to masking the pain often, and we know people really don't want to know how we are feeling so we will not answer that question honestly. Besides, it's impolite to string together a sentence using just swear words when people ask you how you are doing. That is a big difference between people in pain and people in chronic pain. People in pain are permitted to express that pain. They can cry out, limp, or scream. Whatever. People in chronic pain are expected to deal with it, quietly, silently, and without a fuss.

Now, because we are so very good at lying about our pain and are expected to just deal with it, we essentially make our invisible disability more invisible. Pain is not a shared experience. Not only is it something that people have different tolerances for and reactions to, making it a very subjective experience, but we interpret someone else's pain by the behaviors they exhibit.

People can, and do, doubt your pain if you don't exhibit expected physical cues. People may think because you can tolerate pain and work one day that you ought to be able to tolerate pain and work every day. Or people may find it incomprehensible to believe you can be in pain and still smile or laugh, because they wouldn't have the pain tolerance to do so. Others may simply doubt your pain severity and consistency. They may believe you are a chronic complainer, or lazy, or want attention. There is no real way to bridge this gap. As I said, members only. I mean, you could kick the crap out of someone and say, "That's how I feel every day," but you would end up in jail for that bit of communication bridging.

Don't tell someone with chronic pain about some injury you had that lasted for a short time or your occasional "brutal headaches" or that "tennis elbow" that flares up sometimes. Seriously. We may nod and make sympathetic sounds, but really, you've just pissed us off by comparing our constant struggle to your occasional inconvenience. It's not that we don't have sympathy for someone else's pain, it's just that we don't like the comparison.

The lack of an end date gets to all of us eventually. I think it is somewhere after the first decade when you realize it doesn't matter how much you compromise, the pain keeps taking and taking until there is nothing left to take. Somehow you need to think beyond that all-consuming void of pain that lurks in the future, or it will take you. That is our greatest battle. Every day is a battle in the war. And there are victories, but there is no winning. For the long haul though, you have to find things to fill the gaping wounds chronic pain has caused, or the battle may be lost. Doctors treat you as effectively as they know how, given there is no cure and there are limits to how pain can be treated in the long term. They do not, however, treat suffering. You have to define what you can do and what sort of life you can have after grieving for what you had to give up and what is no longer possible. Fill the void with whatever little joys you can in order to survive the war.

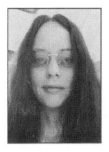 *Nikki Albert is forty years old, living in Alberta, Canada, and lives with a few invisible illnesses. She attained her master of arts in philosophy from the University of Alberta. She enjoys writing fiction and nonfiction as well as blogging. She runs her own blog,* the Brainless Blogger, *and Facebook page,* Making Invisible Disabilities Visible.

That's Why the Lady Was on Stamps

LITSA DREMOUSIS

Seattle, Washington, United States

"YOU SAW THE JOB applications, right?" the social worker asks me and nods in the direction of a bulletin board festooned with red construction paper stars. I imagine the staff meeting where someone asked, "You know what would totally liven this place up and make people forget they're applying for food stamps and other means of government assistance? Stars! Fuck yes, I'll get my tracing paper."

I'm sitting on a gray plastic chair and my crutches are perched against the social worker's battered wooden desk. I reply, "Yes, I saw them," and my voice sounds uncharacteristically timid. She is a woman in her fifties with short brown hair and seems neither kind nor cruel. She briefly makes eye contact before checking a box on the first page of a tall stack of forms. I'm certain she'll forget me by the time I hobble out the sliding glass doors and into the parking lot littered with candy bar wrappers, broken glass, and other debris that somehow didn't make it to the state-issued garbage can perched right there. I need her to remember my case, though, and I feel humiliated and desperate.

It's Seattle, January 2002, and this isn't how I'd planned on starting the new year. But four months prior, I'd experienced a severe relapse of chronic fatigue and immune dysfunction syndrome (CFIDS), an illness that presents in many ways like multiple sclerosis, and I'd found myself in a wheelchair for the second time in a decade. I've progressed to crutches again but am still far too ill to resume work. My money is gone. I was fortunate enough to be born to a family of some means. I attended private schools growing up. My parents have been incredibly supportive emotionally and financially for the past ten years, but my depleted health has also depleted their savings.

By twenty-four, I was in a wheelchair for the first time and dozens of physicians had told me I'd never work again. After protracted physical therapy and tapping inner reserves of near-psychotic tenacity, I'd proven them wrong. I was never asymptomatic and was often intensely ill, but I still managed to write.

The social worker hands me a packet so unwieldy it might hold the entire city's allotment of paperwork. I am bogarting everyone's questionnaires, it seems. "Your doctor will have to fill these out and explain that you're too sick to work," she says. "Then we can proceed. In the meantime, you qualify for emergency aid." She's determining the imminent course of my life with the nonchalance of a barista making decaf instead of regular and I feel even more vulnerable. I try not to take her tone personally; when I was healthy, I'd worked as a domestic violence victim advocate during the day while I wrote at night, so I know what it's like to process big decisions quickly. I'm far more fortunate than the women and men I'd see or, for that matter, these poor, beleaguered children only yards away from me now.

"When do I need to turn everything in?" I ask, and again, emit an unfamiliar voice. If I were meeting me for the first time, I'd never guess I'm, well, me. The longer I'm in this office, the more protective skin I shed.

"The instructions are on the first page, okay?" she responds with finality. She clicks a device behind her desk and the dot matrix-type light above her cubicle advances one digit. I reach for my crutches and she asks, "Do you need help?" She asks more as a way of expediting my exit than offering assistance.

"I'm fine," I say. It's the only lie I've told her during this intake.

Few of my loved ones know I was ever on food stamps. I've had an incurable and degenerative illness for twenty-two years and tend to be open about my health, in part because I have little choice. I usually walk with a cane or with crutches and most days get asked, "What'd you do to your leg?" by misguided if well-meaning strangers when I go for my daily walk, fetch groceries, or hail a cab. I give polite but brief answers by rote and rarely feel off-kilter during these exchanges. Long ago, I decided I wouldn't dwell on CFIDS, but I wouldn't deny it, either. Questions organically arise when interacting with everyone from retail clerks asking if they can carry my potential sartorial purchases, to new lovers inquiring how CFIDS affects my sexual drive. (Note: it doesn't.)

But discussing the period I was on food stamps summons memories I've shared only with those in my inner circle, and very rarely at that. The disdain or outright hostility I frequently encountered from grocery store clerks or from customers in line behind me who scoffed when I paid with the telltale currency still reminds me of how close I came to losing my autonomy and how that possibility lingers. What people who've never fought major illness can't quite understand is that the loss of autonomy can be as terrifying as the symptoms themselves. A few cells revolt and you're now looking at your former, healthy life through a membrane: you can see it, but it remains agonizingly out of reach. Despite your best efforts, you're at the mercy of others just to stay afloat.

The United States House of Representatives is presently considering a whopping $4 billion cut to our nation's food stamp budget. If it passes, roughly four million Americans will get booted from the food stamp program with little or no recourse. Or, you know, food. We can debate budgetary concerns ad nauseam, but it doesn't change the axiomatic fact that food is an unavoidable physical need and basic human right. In a nation with ample food, withholding it is punitive. That's perhaps the most disturbing part of the larger discussion: there are Americans who view themselves as impervious to the possibility of food stamps, convinced their bodies and financial circumstances will stay resolute in the face of disaster. Because, of course, they believe on some level they are impervious to disaster itself. That they've eluded it so far because of some grand action on their part, not through chance. By this metric, those on food stamps must have fucked up big time somewhere along the line, committed some mistake so egregious and irredeemable that food is now an option that can be withheld at the whim of a legislative body, not the sustenance without which carbon-based life forms die.

Such reasoning is so flawed, it would be laughable if its repercussions weren't so destructive. Are there persons who abuse the food stamp system, parasitic jagweeds who commit fraud and think de facto stealing is A-okay? Yes, of course there are. Assholes permeate every part of society and food stamp recipients are no different. Unquestionably, some of them are unlikeable weasels.

But, of course, that isn't the crux here. A large chunk of our elected officials and their constituents can't imagine they could lose their health or their finances, or that the loss of the former will almost always eradicate the latter. They haven't experienced it, so the possibility stays remote, like a tsunami on the news crashing half a world away. Those of us who have nearly drowned know differently.

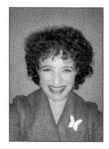

Litsa Dremousis is the author of Altitude Sickness *(Future Tense Books), which Seattle Metropolitan Magazine named one of the all-time "20 Books Every Seattleite Must Read." Her essay "After the Fire" was selected as one of the "Most Notable Essays 2011" by Best American Essays, she's a contributing editor at* The Weeklings, *and* The Seattle Weekly *named her one of "50 Women Who Rock Seattle." She's an essayist with* The Washington Post *and her work appears in a myriad of publications.*

The Things That Go Bump...In Your Body

LINDSEY M. CLOUSER

Wilmington, North Carolina, United States

THERE IS A STRANGE phenomenon that happens when you first get diagnosed with a chronic illness. Some people perceive us as suddenly complaining more or being in more pain. However, that's not what's really happening. It is something that those of us in the chronic illness community discuss very often. When you get diagnosed with a chronic illness, suddenly everything you've been experiencing is made real. We're validated in our pain and suffering. It's a relief, because sometimes we spend years of our lives waiting for that diagnosis, often resulting in person after person, doctor after doctor not believing we're really experiencing anything at all. But it's not the validation that suddenly makes everything seem magnified. It's the fear.

There are very few people who want a chronic illness. I will say, there are some people who enjoy the attention that comes with chronic illnesses. It's these people that make a lot of people doubt us. But most of us hate it. Not only the attention, but the illness itself. Especially if it's an illness that can cause severe damage or eventual disability. Or even worse, already has.

The most common thing doctors tell people with chronic illnesses is that they are unpredictable. That's true. What's also true is that they are downright strange, and most of them are still not completely understood by the medical community. If you're lucky, your diagnosis can explain all your symptoms. In most situations, it can explain some of your symptoms and pain, but doctors will think the rest are side effects that aren't necessarily associated with the illness.

Most people with a chronic illness immediately start to research the illness. Learning everything they can about how it acts, how it progresses, and potential comorbidities. There are very few people diagnosed with a chronic illness that are lucky enough to stay with a single diagnosis. And this magnifies our fears. We're afraid of the progression, the comorbidities. We want to be well. So many of us hope for a diagnosis that will only mean we're in pain. Isn't that sad? We would gladly live with pain if it meant we didn't have to fear damage and debilitation.

This is why we suddenly feel more. It's not that we haven't been experiencing the symptoms. Or the additional pain. It's that we didn't know it could mean something more. Suddenly every pain or extra strange symptom or every bad day could mean the worst in our minds. It could mean something new and bad, or something old and worse. It can be terrifying.

What loved ones should be doing, when our diagnosis magnifies everything, is letting us talk. Let us talk about what's really going on, because we're not looking for attention. We're scared.

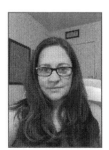

Lindsey M. Clouser lives in Wilmington, North Carolina, with her border collie Davie. She works in finance and in her spare time likes to draw and paint.

The Quandaries of Chronic Pain

ELIN WALTHER

Skåne, Sweden

IN DEALING WITH ANY form of chronic illness, there will be aspects that are difficult. In my case that aspect is the chronic pain. During the past few years I have frequently been asked what it is like to live with this, and I never know how to answer. How do you describe a condition that is so intricate and influences so many facets of your life? Something that's become a major part of who you are?

I have been thinking about this, and have concluded that chronic pain to me, is:

- Difficulty eating, breathing, sleeping, walking, socializing, reading, drawing, exercising, and all the things that should be natural, that should be easy.

- Being chronically fatigued, dizzy, and generally exhausted.

- Spending hours every week on physical therapy despite no recognizable results.

- Seemingly random mood swings throughout the day as pain and energy levels fluctuate.

- Needing to think for an hour before deciding if I can go out.

- Having to cancel plans at the last minute because the pain has become too much.

- Getting exhausted from socializing because of the energy it takes to seem "normal."

- Dreading going to sleep because I know there will be nightmares, sudden jolts of pain, and that I will be in for a world of pain in the morning.

- Having an armory of heating pads, ice packets, muscle tape, joint supports, painkillers, anti-inflammatories, and God knows how many other things in an attempt to manage it all.

- Having to stop and sit down without warning when the vertigo gets too bad.

- Almost falling over on the street when a leg spontaneously decides it does not want to work anymore.

- Dealing with bursts of shooting pain in unpredictable places and patterns.

- Sudden attacks of difficulty breathing from muscle cramps or a flare in pain.

- Falling apart when the pain gets too much to handle, and I feel like I can't keep going.

- Always being prepared for tomorrow to be the worst day yet.

Chronic pain is a lot of things, and I could not possibly sum it all up here. It is difficult, always present, and prevents me from doing a lot of things. However, it is not entirely negative. It is also:

- The reason I have found some of the most amazing people on this planet. Sure, I lost a few on the way. But the ones who stayed are everything anyone could ever ask for, and the ones who left were never worth it to begin with.

- The reason I am strong. I have gotten through everything that has been thrown at me this far, and, with the help of the people I love, I will get through everything that is to come.

- The reason I am me. I have lost who I was before all of this, but I truly believe that who I am now is good enough. Despite the many issues stemming from this illness, I love who I have become.

To everyone that I love, to everyone out there who knows somebody living with this condition, chronic pain does not mean:

- That I don't care. I might zone out occasionally, forget something that you have told me, or just be generally out of it. This has nothing to do with you. I'm trying to keep it all together. Coordinating all the problems from my illness into something semi-normal is a lot of work, but I will always care.

- That I'm not trying. I know it can be frustrating that I can't do everything that you can, that I have to leave early, that I can't come to everything. I wish that I could, and I am always trying my very best.

- That I don't love you. I might get irritable. I might snap at you. I never mean to, and it never means that I do not love you. I love every single one of you so, so much, and I am endlessly grateful that you put up with me and help me with all of this.

Please be patient. Talk to me, ask me questions, and ask how I am doing. I may not always be clear about what is happening, but I will always appreciate you caring to ask. I want you to understand, but it is not always an easy thing to explain. For anyone interested in understanding better, look up the "Spoon Theory."[7]

---

7 Spoon Theory is a concept developed by Christine Miserandino and fully explained on her website at butyoudontlooksick.com. "Spoons"

While this may not apply to everybody, I have found that simply showing this article to people in my life who wonder about chronic illness has been a massive help in giving them perspective.

To all of you out there dealing with some type of chronic illness, it is going to be a long ride, and it will be difficult. But you can do it. Find your coping strategies, find your people, and hug your dog. You can be happy despite all of it, and I hope everything goes well for every single one of you. Love and spoons to you all.

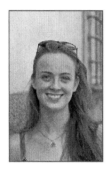 *Elin Walther is a twenty-year-old living with fibromyalgia, Raynaud's syndrome, and joint hypermobility syndrome. She loves video games, her two dogs, and updating her friends with spontaneous observations about odd things that happen in her day. She chooses to believe they love it much more than they actually do. She is currently working toward a bachelor's degree in development studies at Lund University.*

---

is often used as shorthand for the available capacity to manage fatigue and other symptoms of chronic illness.

A Little Understanding

MARY LEE EVELYN KEENEY
Baltimore, Maryland, United States

I WISH THAT MORE people would take chronic invisible ill-nesses seriously—especially chronic migraines. I have been suf-fering for eleven years without a successful treatment. I have exhausted nearly every treatment option available to me, and so far, nothing has worked. My illness is not allowing me to have an acceptable quality of life.

People with chronic migraines are often labeled as lazy or anti-social. But who wants to be in a room full of people when you have a full-blown migraine? It makes socializing difficult. It makes working difficult. We often lose our jobs and friends. Family members don't understand. We may lock ourselves in a dark, quiet room for hours or days at a time. But we didn't choose this, and we are suffering.

I am in pain all the time, with a migraine every day; if I tell you that I cannot do something, please believe me. Ignoring my pain to hold a conversation is exhausting. I may have put on a fake smile all day at work, so when you ask me to hang out, the answer might be no. I might just want to curl up in a blanket and forget how to be a person for a while. My relationships suffer. I have lost a lot of friends because I am no longer able to keep in touch. For those who think texting is not good enough, it might be all we have. If I am unable to get out of bed, at least I braved the brightness of my phone screen and the stabbing pains in the back of my head it will cause to let you know that I'm thinking of you.

If we ask you to do something, please do not fight with us about it. Know that when I ask you to drive me somewhere, it's because I no longer trust my own eyes. I know that you may be tired, but my vision is wavy and none of the lines on the road will stay still. Please don't tell me that because I drove earlier, that I can drive now. My symptoms can change from one second to the next. And I really don't want to get into another car accident.

When talking to someone with chronic illness, please, if you can help it, try to avoid using phrases like, "When you get better," or "When you're cured." We may never be cured. We may never get better. That's why our illnesses are called chronic. They are ongoing with no end in sight. We have good and bad days. Instead say, "When you're having a good day," or "When this flare is over." That might give us some short-term hope that on our next good day we'll have something fun to do. I have had people tell me, "When you get better, maybe you won't have to take all those pills." I don't expect to be getting better; my disease has been getting progressively worse for three years. These phrases are just a reminder that I will never get back to how healthy I once was.

If you know someone who has chronic migraines or any other chronic illness, don't treat them like a problem to be solved. Just because your sister cured her arthritis with eucalyptus leaves and oils does not mean that it will work for me. If every time we see each other you bring new information about how aromatherapy, yoga, or even a piercing will help me, we will stop hanging out. Don't tell me what to do with my body and my health unless I explicitly ask you. You may mean well, but I am not a problem to be solved, and you are not my doctor.

There is a lot of stigma attached to migraines as a chronic illness. I've needed to convince people too many times that I am not drunk or high or spacing out, I have severe brain fog. The brain controls every little thing about your body, and when it is diseased or doesn't work right, just about anything can go wrong. Those of us with chronic migraines are fighting a battle against our own brain and all we really want is a little understanding. A migraine is never just a headache.

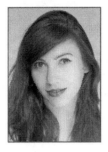

Mary Lee is a twenty-something Baltimore native and a passionate patient advocate. A chronic pain patient with a degree in fine arts, she uses her experiences to create. Her hobbies include anything from photography and design to spending time with her dogs.

Part 7

Others' Perceptions

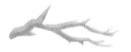

No Different from Anyone Else

GLYNIS SCRIVENS

Brisbane, Queensland, Australia

IT'S BEEN AN EYE-OPENER for me, viewing the world from a wheel-chair. I'm used to the anonymity of walking, something you just take for granted until it's taken away from you. Once you're sitting in a wheelchair, you force everyone else to decide. How will they behave when they pass you?

You can see the indecision written on their faces, even from ten meters away. Averting eyes is the simplest option, but it causes guilt. There but for the grace of God, they're thinking. Do they say hello?

The problem with saying hello is that they need to physically look down on you, and that causes them to feel awkward too. A good compromise is when they can say hello to my husband, who's pushing me. That skirts the issue nicely. To make it easier I smile at them. Just a small "I'm okay" sort of smile, nothing that invades their personal space or demands a response. But mostly it's a bit of a no-win situation punctuated by awkwardness. For adults, that is. I always get happy responses from young children when they cross paths with my chair. "Ah, an adult, this is fun," they're thinking. It's a revelation to them.

I guess the fun part for me is getting in and out of the chair and seeing the startled reactions. People seem to believe you either need a chair 100 percent of the time, or not at all. Finding somebody in-between pushes them out of their comfort zone. Shops are the places you see this most. Picture it: my husband wheels me around a shopping mall. We reach an interesting shop, and out I get. Walking about to explore. Jaws drop. People can't help staring. Escalators go the same way. I just stand up, and for those few moments I look like everyone else. People look at me as if I'm advertising a miracle cure.

My younger daughter has instructed me before, "When you're in the chair, stay in it. You can't be getting in and out." She wasn't sure how her colleagues at work would react once they'd seen me in the chair, to then have to readjust their thinking. People like to put you in a box in their mind, stick on a label. Someone who doesn't fit into one of their boxes isn't appreciated. It's as if they feel they've been tricked into feeling sorry for you.

Occasionally you find genuine understanding. It's rare, so it's treasured. In the hectic pre-Christmas rush, we went to a big department store. One lovely shop assistant simply asked me, "What have you done to yourself?" A simple direct question, asked with compassion. It turned out she suffered from multiple sclerosis. Perhaps there are occasions when she too needs to use a chair, I wonder. Some shop assistants automatically speak to my husband, even in newsstands when I'm the one holding the magazines.

It's summer in Brisbane. My husband wheels me through the beautiful tranquil avenues in South Bank every other day for a swim in one of the pools. My empty chair by the pool arouses curiosity. Looking on, no one can tell which one of us in the water has mobility problems. It's nice to regain my anonymity here, for a time at least.

Next time you see someone in a wheelchair, just treat them like you would any other person—because that's exactly who we are.

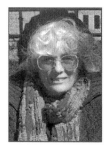

Glynis Scrivens is an Australian writer of short stories and magazine articles. Her book Edit is a Four-Letter Word *includes what she has learned about the writing process. Glynis lives in Brisbane, Queensland, Australia, with her family, two dogs, a Himalayan Persian called Mr. Floof, nine chickens, three ducks, and goldfish. She can be found at glynisscrivens.com.*

Chronic Pain Versus Masculinity

BRET STEPHENSON

Reno, Nevada, United States

I HAVE A TENDENCY to reflect on my path through chronic pain over the three decades I've been dealing with it. A gifted athlete, adventurous, I liked to play hard and have a lot of fun. Ironically, I never hurt my back.

Decade one was my thirties. I did pretty well managing to get through most of what I had been doing back then, but now I have much more soreness over the following few days, or longer. I was living in Lake Tahoe, Nevada, with tough winters that required moving a lot of snow, prepping lots of firewood, and other preparations of long winters. As a man, I wanted and needed to do these things, but they were getting increasingly harder. I started to learn how to swallow that male pride and ask for more help with certain things, each time feeling less of a man. Men take care of business. Heck, we can't even ask for directions when traveling at the risk of looking weak and lacking control.

In my forties, my back got much worse. I spent thousands of dollars trying to keep it healthy and functional. My wife had to clean out the rain gutters as I had trouble with ladders and reaching above my head. Everyone had a bad back story to share, and a cure to try that had helped them that one time they strained their back. I was wearing back and shoulder braces, getting weekly massages, acupuncture, too much chiropractic work, and trying everything else I could find. Doctors gave me pain pills, anti-inflammatories, and muscle relaxants. I found myself thankful my golden retriever wasn't a fetch addict like my last one, as throwing sticks and balls was getting harder each year.

I wasted money on new mattress systems, desperate for a decent night's sleep. Sitting on the ground, on the beach, on my mountain bike, in my canoe—all got more and more difficult with longer recovery time. I felt like a wimp, and more often than not I was saying, "No thanks" to my friends' invitations to golf, water ski, backpack, or even sit on the deck and have a few beers. Pretty soon, they quit calling.

I retreated into less-manly activities like sitting in a soft chair to read, use my laptop, or sleep. I was an adolescent counselor, and I used teen labor more and more often as I became unable to move my furniture around, do landscaping, or shovel snow. Road trips and other travel dwindled as I struggled with strange sleeping arrangements, painful travel, and then what to do when I got to my destination. By then, I knew I had fibromyalgia, arthritis, and muscle atrophy. Doctors were still working on the rest of my symptoms.

Annual trips to southern California every Thanksgiving to visit my father-in-law included Disneyland trips with my young daughter; I loved it. I'd grit my teeth when I put her on my shoulders so she could see the closing parade better. The next year my wife did the shoulder thing while I stood helpless, ready to leave, but unwilling to say so. Then I had to sit and rest while my daughter and wife played, saving my energy for the rides and activities I most wanted to do, or could do. No more wild rides that jarred this failing body. After a few more years I stopped going at all, unable to walk Disneyland anymore and unwilling, "as a man," to use a wheelchair and be subjected to pity stares. Thus, I had to settle for the stories brought back to me after a day of vegging out on the couch feeling useless and less than a man, as well as a poor dad.

Then my fifties hit, and it all went south from there. Finally diagnosed with congenital canal stenosis, I've now had three back and neck fusions and carry around a couple dozen pieces of titanium in my back holding it all together. Disregarding all the rehab time, my quality of life continued to decline. Going to a restaurant or not was now based on their seating softness. One-day road trips became two-day trips so I could rest, and my wife did most of the driving while I took pain pills and Valium and tried not to break everything in sight from frustration and pain.

I regained some self-respect after much hard work after the first two fusions. I could ride a bike for half an hour, swim laps, and walk a mile or two if necessary. I managed a few scuba dives, enjoying the weightlessness of the water. I could even shoot a few baskets with my teen clients or throw the baseball around. Woven into this progress, though, was necessary downtime for me to recover from the previous day's exploits. I could take a hike in the Utah Canyonlands with my wife and daughter, then had to send them off by themselves the next day while I rested. Camping stopped as I could not find a way to sleep on the ground. My wife ended up taking my daughter camping and I'd make day trips out to join them, then go home to a less-than-comfortable bed. I began sleeping in my recliner more often, and now I live in it. I don't even own a bed.

The list goes on. Then a handful of years after the success of the first two surgeries, the stenosis moved again, necessitating a third fusion that was brutal to rehab at almost sixty years old. Shortly after returning to work, my back would not get better and actually seemed to be declining again. Two neurosurgeons, a psychiatrist, and an orthopedic surgeon all had different ideas as to what might be going on but no one offered any concrete solutions. So I kept enduring.

After almost a year and a half of expecting another surgery of some kind, I received good and bad news. The good news was there was nothing surgically to fix. The bad news was there was nothing surgically to fix. I got a new, fancy term to explain my situation: post-laminectomy syndrome. In English that means my back is beat to shit after three surgeries and thirty years of chronic pain. Fibromyalgia, arthritis, muscle atrophy, nerve damage, and scar tissue all together make me feel like someone hit me in the lower back with a bat, or I gardened for three days bent over.

Now my battered masculinity and manhood are dealing with being on Social Security Disability Insurance[8] and unable to work. Like many men, much of my identity is attached to what I do—working with high-risk teens. I like what I do and don't like how people now perceive me as retired. Plus, trying to survive on 40 percent of what I made a year ago has me groveling to family members for money and getting friends to do simple things like moving a piece of furniture or a box of books.

Now sixty and allegedly an elder, I'm treated like the world wants to put me out to pasture. I've never agreed with the concept of retirement, a modern invention that separates elders from the youngsters we are supposed to teach, as well as continuing to fragment the extended family problems in America. Women now open doors for me, which I do appreciate, but part of me remains chivalrous and wants to open it for them. I was embarrassed the past two years while working in Prague (don't even ask about the travel challenges) when old women offered me their seats on the tram. My pride and ego constantly argued with the need to get off my feet for a few minutes, while watching someone's grandma hang onto the rails.

I can no longer afford the apartment I have and am getting a roommate to cut my expenses. I feel like I'm back in college,

---

8 Social Security Disability Insurance is a government benefit in the United States that some with disabilities are eligible to apply for.

almost forty years ago, broke and playing roommate, asking my eighty-seven-year-old father for money. My ego is pretty bruised. I've had to pull my IRA retirement money for medical bills three times, leaving it empty with no cushion to fall back on. This creates a fear of failure more than a fear of poverty—the failure part of my clinging attempt to feel like a self-sufficient man.

What I have learned through all of this is my masculinity, my manhood, must be malleable like my overall pride. They all become a luxury at a certain point, with necessity dictating when to bend and adapt. Part of my personal growth has been to stop fighting my back issues like a man "should," and just let go of any expectations from my body. A local chronic pain group helps, but it took me months to swallow my male pride and walk through the door. The few guys who show, much outnumbered by women, have expressed many of the same feelings as their own personal abilities and dreams were altered by chronic pain. The strong male oak must become a flexible willow.

Men do not have to take pain and challenges stoically, especially when they simply cannot. We must let go of all those age-old stereotypes and expectations. We need to not get angry when our friends complain of a sore back after golfing or hiking; it's a poor attempt to commiserate but an attempt nonetheless. Using a cane or butt-cushion is not a sign of weakness, just adaptation. Leaving a group early because you can't sit any longer is not a sign of weakness, nor is pulling the social plug completely some days to just try and get through the day and night.

I have little to prove as a man at this point in my life. Rather, I've let go of my old manhood and masculinity dogma, and my new goal is to ride this out gracefully and hopefully with a sense of humor.

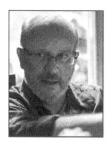

Before back and neck problems forced Bret onto disability benefits, he specialized in high-risk teenagers for almost thirty years, particularly gang youth. Three back and neck fusions unfortunately pulled him out of that work, but he keeps a few projects going through the pain. Bret is the author of From Boys to Men: Spiritual Rites of Passage in an Indulgent Age *and* The Undercurrents of Adolescence: Tracking the Evolution of Modern Adolescence and Delinquency Through Classic Cinema. *After twenty-six years in Lake Tahoe, Nevada, Bret is back in his hometown of Reno, Nevada, to get out of the snow!*

The Importance of Representation: Why Using My First Cane Was Scary

REBECCA BARTLETT

Crete, Nebraska, United States

TAYLOR SWIFT'S SONG "22" was released right before I turned twenty-two years old. If you haven't heard it, it describes the singer's wish to act like a woman in her early twenties: having a good time with her lover while going to parties, staying up all night, and goofing off. Well, the year I turned twenty-two years old was also the year I started using a cane for mobility.

I avoided using my cane in college because I felt so shy about it. It's one thing to use the cane on shopping trips with my family and friends, who love me unconditionally. But it's quite another to use it around people who don't know about my disability and might say something ignorant or even cruel. They may have never met someone as young as me using a cane before, and so they might not know what to do.

When I was twenty-four years old, I had graduated and gotten a full-time job. After three weeks of rain, which were not so great for my joints, I needed to use my cane quite a bit in front of my new colleagues. I've learned a lot from that. Most of the people in my office completely ignored my awkward journey to and from the elevator. Those I worked closely with asked what happened, thinking I had gotten into an accident of some sort, and I explained that I have joint pain when the weather is bad. Their responses ranged from simple apologies and well wishes to awkward mumbling.

There's one instance of awkwardness that really stands out in my mind as the moment when I stopped feeling weird about other people's responses. A man was exiting the restroom, which was across the hall from the women's restroom that I was headed for, and when he saw me heading toward him with a cane he started to hold the door open for me. He then turned bright red as he realized that I was not headed into that room and quickly walked past me. I was very careful not to laugh because his heart was in the right place.

Back when I was still in college, I took a psychology class where we learned about cognitive dissonance. The dictionary definition from Merriam-Webster is, "Psychological conflict resulting from incongruous beliefs and attitudes held simultaneously." The way our professor explained it was that if you walked into a bar and saw a cowboy knitting, you'd probably have cognitive dissonance because there are a certain set of beliefs you have about the things cowboys do, and a separate set of beliefs about people who knit, and those likely do not match up. I cause people cognitive dissonance when I use my cane. Like Taylor Swift sings in her song "22," most people have a set of beliefs about what women in their twenties do and are like, and those ideas don't include being differently-abled.

Is this right or wrong? Well, it's kind of both. Most twenty-somethings aren't disabled, so it's a valid generalization. A little bit of cognitive dissonance doesn't hurt. I would guess most people simply go through a process of thinking, "Huh, that's odd that she has joint pain at a young age, but I guess it happens. It's not really my business," or something similar, and that's all it takes to solve their cognitive dissonance.

But, now consider those who don't believe disabilities exist. That is too much dissonance. People who claim pain is "all in your head" or say a panic attack is "asking for attention" have too much dissonance. These are people who cannot solve or fathom these conflicting ideas, and so they simply choose to believe the other person is lying.

Raising awareness about disabilities by writing articles, creating art, and simply living life demonstrates to others that disabilities are valid and destigmatizes them. This helps minimize instances of cognitive dissonance. Colleges are beginning to see clubs such as the Student Occupational Therapy Association, or general disability awareness groups open on their campuses. Other campuses and communities are celebrating weeks or months dedicated to disability awareness. For younger students, both the Boy Scouts of America and the Girl Scouts of America have created merit badges related to disability awareness. Creating awareness can be done in many forms, and every bit helps remind others that there is always more to learn.

Maybe Taylor Swift isn't going to write a song about a twenty-two-year-old who doesn't sleep because the pain keeps her up, and who leaves parties early because her medications won't allow her to drink, but that's okay. With the recent advances in destigmatization there are now more allies, and more allies means better treatment from others and fewer awkward moments. And we could all do with fewer awkward moments.

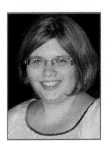

Rebecca Bartlett has a degree in English and has worked in journalism and freelance writing. In her free time, Rebecca enjoys writing poetry, playing video games, and volunteering. She lives in Nebraska with her fiancé and husky mix.

Hope's Visible in Me: How My Invisible Illness Is Actually Visible

JESSICA WARD

Newark, New York, United States

PEOPLE LIKE TO CALL my chronic illnesses and disabilities "invisible." I'm still not sure why; perhaps it's to downplay the seriousness of these conditions, or perhaps it's to somehow encourage me in a weird, twisted way. I can understand where the label is coming from, really, I can. It's clear that Crohn's disease isn't as visible as, say, cancer. You wouldn't look at me and be able to see I had fibromyalgia or autonomic nervous system dysfunction. Asthma isn't visible because you can't see my lungs. And I get it, I really do. But despite all these (very valid) arguments, my illnesses are visible. If you look closely, you can see.

If you look at my hair, you'll see the dull color and thinning strands. Thanks to years of dehydration, malnutrition, and vitamin deficiencies, I've kissed healthy hair goodbye. So long Rapunzel. Prednisone, chemo drugs, and maintenance medications have given me a more Tinkerbell-like head.

If you look at my arms, you'll see greens, blues, purples, and yellows. I don't have tattoos. I have bruises from infiltrated intravenous fluids, painful unsuccessful blood draws, and blood thinning medications. I like to think I'm walking art, but I just look like I'm searching for my next high.

If you look at my eyes, you'll see dilated pupils from pain medications I need to get through some days. Glazed over baby blues with a trace of cynicism and a large amount of pain, searching for something hopeful to hold onto—those are mine.

If you look at my body, you'll see stretch marks from weight loss and weight gain. Acne from steroids, rashes from allergic reactions, scars from days that I didn't want to live anymore. They're all there and painfully visible.

My diseases aren't invisible. Crohn's disease is visible in my scars and steroid-induced moon face. Gastroparesis is visible in my bloated tummy and skinny wrists. Fibromyalgia is visible in my slow, crooked gait. Postural orthostatic tachycardia syndrome is visible in my purple hands and pale skin. Chronic migraines are visible in my squinted eyes.

But more than the illnesses themselves, hope is visible. It's visible in getting out of bed every morning, even to just change pajamas and get cozy again. It's visible in the smiles that break free, even during ambulance rides. Hope is visible in taking another breath, and trying to eat again. It's visible in having a Super Bowl party after a hospital admission. It's visible in jokes said before surgeries.

Hope is visible in me.

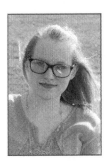

Jessica Ward is a twenty-something lover of coffee, art, and history. She is learning how to thrive while living with chronic illness.

High-Maintenance

LINDSEY M. CLOUSER
Wilmington, North Carolina, United States

I NEVER REALIZED HOW much ableism had been instilled in me by society and my upbringing until I began living with multiple chronic illnesses. I was diagnosed with my first chronic illness when I was six years old and began collecting them from there. I have always had to make small adjustments here and there, but when I was diagnosed with psoriatic arthritis it was the straw that broke the camel's back. I had to control every aspect of my life. At this time, the chronic illness affected my skin, my musculoskeletal system, my gastrointestinal system, and my brain. I had to control what I ate, how much I ate, skin care, exercise, daily activities, and sleep. Not a single corner of my life remained untouched. Even my poor dog has had to adjust; I'm sad to say playing tug of war with him is no longer an option.

A few months after being diagnosed with psoriatic arthritis, I took a long weekend to go visit my sister and mom. I used to be a very light packer; I needed very little to go away for a few days. When I began packing I realized how much I now needed in order to remain in a good place. I had become so sensitive to temperature that I needed more clothing to ensure I remained at the right temperature. I had so many more medications and supplements. The bag that used to hold everything I needed for a weekend was now filled to the brim with only the "just in case" materials I needed. Extra medication if I had a high pain day, wrist guards to ensure I didn't accidentally hurt my wrists and hands while I slept, ear plugs for if I had a high sound sensitivity day, a yoga mat for if I needed to stretch out my back, and extra wraps for my hands and feet if I overexerted myself. I could go on.

I even found my behavior different once I joined my sister and mom. I was so concerned that my actions could result in a flare-up. I was going out of my way to hydrate. I volunteered to do the grocery shopping to ensure we had healthy food available. I even volunteered to cook and showed up with desserts that wouldn't cause a migraine or flare-up. I took precautions in every aspect. My family certainly noticed. After just a day my sister made the comment, "Wow, you've become very high-maintenance." And there it was.

I wonder at what point in my life "high-maintenance" had become an insult. I can't pinpoint it, but it certainly felt like a slap in the face. All my life I'd been programmed to be easy going, independent, resourceful, and not bother anyone. Even as a child I wouldn't complain when I didn't feel well. All my life when I've been sad or in a bad mood I would withdraw instead of upsetting someone. It had clearly become very ingrained that I shouldn't bother other people. But now I was high-maintenance, and it upset me. The worst part was, I wasn't asking for anything. I never asked for help. I carried my own bags, I carried the groceries, I cooked, I chopped vegetables, and I helped take care of my nephew. I didn't ask for any help at all. In fact, I was contributing to the collective, yet I was being pegged as high-maintenance. Why on earth should this bother me, and why would taking better care of myself cause my mom and sister to strap me with this horrible attribute? Why does this automatically feel like such a bad attribute?

The problem with the term high-maintenance is that so many of us associate it with selfishness. It's perceived as needing others to take care of you with a great amount of effort, of putting your needs above others and asking them to do the same. At least, this is how I perceive high-maintenance. In truth, high-maintenance is just that: one who requires a lot of maintenance. It's true that some people just require more maintenance. Our systems are more delicate and sensitive. We need certain conditions in order to be okay and certain supports so that we may function. This is not something we can control. Yet so many of us are raised to present ourselves as the opposite: as low-maintenance, strong people who don't need anything. That anything further is simply a burden on our family and friends, or on society. Which is just ridiculous. I am very lucky in that right now, I can provide my own maintenance. I very rarely need to ask for assistance. But it might not always be that way. My need to take care of myself in such a thorough way is my attempt at preventing myself from becoming a drain on others.

It really struck me that my mom and sister should already understand. They both have at least two chronic illnesses each. Of all the people in the world to suddenly judge me on this, I thought they would understand. Don't they have to take care of themselves too? That's how I realized that I'm the only one in my family who practices active self-care. This absolutely blew my mind. They both have chronic illnesses and yet, they don't take proper care of themselves. Instead they take the role of caretaker and put themselves last. I understand there will be times that come up where we put ourselves second and prioritize the collective over the individual. But why would the other women in my family not take care of themselves?

I've realized the reason high-maintenance felt like such an insult is because that's what society and our families have always taught us to feel. That we're supposed to put ourselves last and the collective first. That women should be caregivers, not need care. By practicing self-care, I was allowing my family to see that I have needs and that I'm willing to meet those needs myself.

Because I am a woman, and a member of a family, and continue to prioritize myself and my well-being, I'm perceived as selfish.

Prioritizing the self-care makes sense. I recognize that by taking care of myself now, it is less likely for me to become dependent on others later. I need to minimize the damage these chronic illnesses do to my body where I can. The care I give myself also allows me to contribute to the family. In my mind, how am I ever supposed to care for others or contribute to others if I don't also take care of myself? This is the reality of life. If I don't care for myself, I will become dependent on care from others later in life.

Society has created unrealistic expectations of us all. They expect us to be low-maintenance for all our lives and never be a drain on others, all the while taking care of those who need us. It's taught us to look down on those who need help. Well, that's just crap. Society needs to adapt. We are all different, we all have different needs, and we all can contribute in different ways. Just because some of us contribute less, doesn't make that contribution less amazing. If we all practiced self-care, maybe we would put more value on those differences, on understanding, and on compassion.

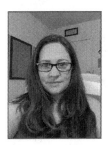

Lindsey M. Clouser lives in Wilmington, North Carolina, with her border collie Davie. She works in finance and in her spare time likes to draw and paint.

We Don't Get Any Medals

JANE LESLEY

Newcastle upon Tyne, United Kingdom

I'VE BEEN ILL ON and off ever since I got measles as a very tiny baby. From then on, I've had many surgeries and many chronic illnesses. I have two kinds of people in my life: those who empathize; and those who want to find an answer, a reason why I am sick on a particular occasion with yet another illness. The people in the latter group blame me, the victim.

They don't realize they're doing it. They're not being unkind. They want me to be well, and want to believe the illness is under my control so that they can worry less about the arbitrary nature of my health issues. Just the other day, a friend told me that she'd been talking to her sister-in-law about my latest illness and passed on to me that her response had been, "I just don't believe how Jane can get all those illnesses." She meant to be empathic, but her choice of words was interesting.

Here's the litany: Crohn's disease; degenerative disc disease; disembarkment syndrome (a rare disease affecting balance); depression; and a history of adenomyosis, gallstones, torn ligament, migraines, asthma, anosmia, malaria, and bilateral pulmonary emboli—to name a few. With practically every sickness, atypical symptoms lead to a diagnosis of, "It's all in your head," until another doctor well-read in the particular illness figures it out.

I suspect I'm preaching to the choir here, especially if you're female and over forty, because then you know firsthand that we are prone to exaggerate pain. Or at least that's what some young doctors seem to have been taught. My mother used to say, when a doctor patronized her, "sexism and ageism." Sometimes she even said it to the doctor. I was very proud of her when she did.

Do I sound bitter and angry? I think I am this morning. Usually I'm a pretty good patient, with a good sense of humor. I tend to underreport, rather than overreport, my health challenges. I am proactive. I have developed a good team of doctors who *get* me.

Just once, though, I'd like someone to say, "You really cope well with adversity." Not because I need compliments, so much as I would like to feel seen as the courageous woman I have had to be. I suspect that here in this anthology, there will be many courageous men and women who are the unsung heroes. The ones who get up every day and fight a battle with pain and illness and who don't get any medals for it.

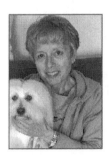 *Jane Lesley is a retired social worker living in Newcastle, United Kingdom. She has been living with Crohn's disease for over forty years but has moved her home between three continents nonetheless.*

My Journey for Answers: Because No One Will Care More about My Health Than Me

JULIE MORGENLENDER

Concord, Massachusetts, United States

THE SYMPTOMS STARTED WHEN I was twelve years old, but we had no idea what they were symptoms of. The wrist pain would appear sporadically and resolve after a few weeks of wearing splints. The doctors kept saying that it was tendonitis even though it clearly was not. We didn't know then that it would be eleven years before I would get my first correct diagnosis. By that time, I had been in pain for half my life.

When I was sixteen, the pain changed. It became more intense, and constant. Suddenly, I was in pain every second of every day. I remember driving to work one day about nine years later, sitting at a stoplight and suddenly realizing that I could not remember what it felt like to not be in pain. Despite the overwhelming sadness I felt when I realized that, I had to pull myself together and go to work. That's how I managed; I survived my life with chronic illness by compartmentalizing, and there was no room for devastating sadness when I had to get to my job.

For a long time, I saw a lot of doctors without receiving any answers. One doctor told me to stop coming in because nobody could help me. I gave up for a long time after that. I pushed through the pain and graduated from high school while working, worked more jobs and graduated from college, got an exploratory surgery that only made things worse, worked a full-time job, and then went to graduate school while working two jobs. It was in graduate school that I decided to address the pain again.

I was struggling a lot. And it wasn't just the pain in my wrists now. The pain that had started in my wrists when I was twelve had spread to my knees in college. The digestive problems that had been labeled irritable bowel syndrome (IBS) continued, and doctors stuck with the diagnosis even though the symptoms didn't match the description of IBS. The fatigue that started after I got a mono-like virus in college and had never fully resolved, continued. At times I was scared. Part of me had accepted that I would always be in pain, while another part wanted to fight back, to make the pain stop. As I teenager I had learned to sleep through all but the worst of the pain, otherwise I wouldn't sleep. Many days I could not hold a pen, use a can opener, or lift anything more than a few pounds. I struggled, but what else could I do?

In graduate school I found myself in a unique position: I was able to get back on my parents' insurance because I was a student (a necessity, back before Obamacare), while I was also on the university's less comprehensive insurance. My parents' insurance in Massachusetts said that because I was living out of state, I could see any doctor who would submit the proper forms for reimbursement, and they would cover me. I decided to take advantage of that because for the first time in my life, I did not need a referral to see a specialist. Not needing a referral made all the difference.

Joint pain was still my only "real" symptom. In our society, fatigue is just something you deal with because everyone gets tired, right? And the gastrointestinal problems had been labeled IBS and so I felt I should just deal with it. But the joint pain was something everyone agreed was abnormal—at least, the folks who believed me. In all of those years of pain, many people, including doctors, said the pain was all in my head. When I was younger, I was told I was only saying I had pain in order to get attention. I wish I could bring my staggering list of diagnoses, including secondary conditions due to damage from too many years of being untreated, to those disbelieving doctors.

Sitting in the linguistics department's computer lab and looking up joint pain, I found the Arthritis Foundation's website and learned I should be seeing a rheumatologist. I had been referred to a rheumatologist once before, for a single visit six years prior. The doctor told me that the test showed I did not have lupus. This was shocking to me because no one had ever told me they were testing me for lupus. My mother was with me at that appointment, as she was with me at almost all appointments because, remember, I was only a teenager. I could not even drive yet. She had no idea they were testing me for lupus either. Supposedly they had not wanted to worry to me. But this meant we hadn't prepared the right questions to ask the doctor. Once he said that I did not have lupus, my other doctors didn't want to refer me to a rheumatologist again. What a loss. Six years later I referred myself to a rheumatologist and it changed my life.

At the first appointment, he told me that he was pretty sure I had autoimmune connective tissue disease, but he wanted to run tests to be certain. Sure enough, the tests showed that I had autoimmune disease. In fact, he found in my records that the same test he ran that day had come back abnormally high three times in the past. It was not previously high enough to confirm autoimmune disease, but high enough that the results should have been flagged and followed, but that hadn't happened. This fourth time the test levels were high enough that I clearly had autoimmune disease. It had been years since that test had last been run and I wonder how much sooner I could have been diagnosed if my doctors had followed up on it. In fact, with the previous high test results and my symptoms, I probably could have been diagnosed much sooner, but these latest tests made it clear.

The diagnosis was undifferentiated connective tissue disease. If that sounds odd to you, that's because it is. It basically meant that I had an autoimmune disease but that they couldn't classify it. There wasn't, and still isn't, enough information about these diseases. That meant that I didn't know what it was. Friends and family who meant well tried to tell me that one day research would give me the answer. I tried to explain that it simply isn't being funded. Maybe one day there will be an answer, but I don't know if that will be in my lifetime. It has already been almost twenty years since that diagnosis with no additional answers.

I was hugely relieved to finally have a diagnosis. I was also devastated, because this was now real. I couldn't pretend it was all some strange mistake that would go away. I had already gone through the five stages of grief as a teenager dealing with constant pain, but following this diagnosis—this new loss—I went through them again.

The rheumatologist told me to avoid stress and I laughed, because doesn't everyone have stress? But eventually I realized he was right. Graduate school was too much of a strain. Everything was difficult and painful, and causing symptoms that I couldn't even put into words. I remember crying one day from the effort of heating up a can of soup on the stove. Just carrying the bowl to the table was too much for me. I spoke to my advisor and arranged to get my degree one term earlier than planned. I missed Boston, so I came back, moved in with my parents, and rested for about six weeks before I looked for a job. I probably needed a lot more rest. When I got to their house, I literally felt like I was dying, like my life energy was being drained from me. But I pushed through because that is what you do, right? I didn't know any other way. Thankfully, this past year, at the age of thirty-nine,

I began working with a therapist who has experience working with chronic illness patients. I am now learning how to better handle the grief and frustration of chronic illness. But back then, I didn't have these tools and pushing through was all I knew.

After several years of working full time, I was struggling with pain, fatigue, and other symptoms I couldn't put a name to. The pain had spread to more of my joints. After putting it off for far too long, I had finally gotten an accessible parking placard. It was very emotional to admit I needed that placard, but it helped. I would sometimes wake up in the morning feeling so exhausted that I couldn't even reach for the phone on my nightstand to call into work and say I would be late. I finally arranged with my boss to work from home one day per week. This made a huge difference. I still struggled a lot, but it helped. I began to take short walks, despite the fatigue. I started with a very slow five-minute walk up the street and then back home, and over time I was able to increase it to fifteen minutes. It was small, but at least it was an improvement.

Then one day when I was in my mid-twenties, I tried a disease-modifying drug that reduced the pain, and I was shocked. I still had pain, but for the first time in nine-and-a-half years I had a moment without pain. I was able to remember what it felt like to not be in pain, or at least to not be aware of the pain. I still have moments without pain and I am incredibly grateful for that. They don't last long, and in truth there is probably pain somewhere in my body, but I've gotten very good at ignoring any pain that is less severe. Either way, I am grateful for it.

When I left that job, I unexpectedly took a year off. I had been working since I was a teenager and it felt really good to stop working. Of course, that wasn't my intent. I had already been interviewing for new jobs, but I decided to quit the old job before I found a new one because I was so miserable. Then I thought I would take a few weeks off. And that turned into a few months. And that turned into a few more months. I waited six months before I even began looking for work again. I was simply burnt out. During that time, I finally got into the habit of exercising regularly, doing my physical therapy almost daily, learning how to cook properly, and eating more healthy foods. I am so grateful I learned how to cook during that time, because a few years later it became much more necessary.

When I went back to work, I got a job with shorter hours, a simple nine-to-five, and I thought that would make up for not being able to work from home anymore. I was wrong. I struggled a lot, and things continued to get worse. To manage a bout of severe pain I had to go on prednisone, not for the first time. But this time I just could not get off of it. It is important to slowly taper down the dose before stopping prednisone, and every time I reduced the dose below five milligrams I had a horrible flare of symptoms. It took a long time before I was finally off of it.

Once off the prednisone, my fatigue returned with a vengeance. Every morning I would have to lay down and rest for twenty minutes in the middle of getting dressed because I was so exhausted. I arrived at work feeling like I was already ready to go to sleep and the day had not even started. I had to stop taking the subway to work and instead drive the two miles, even though traffic was horrible and it took me half an hour each way. I simply did not have the energy to walk to and from the subway stops as I had only weeks prior. I would get home from work every day and have to rest for an hour or two before I had the energy to eat dinner. I would then spend the rest of the night watching TV. I simply did not have the energy to do anything else, even though I wanted to. I had to stop going out with friends during the week. Finally, I spoke to my rheumatologist and asked if she would write a letter for me to take a leave of absence from work for two months. She gently suggested I make it three months. I think she knew at that point that I would not be going back, but was trying to ease me into it. We had previously discussed the possibility of me no longer being able to work, but I had assumed that was still years away. After three months, though, I felt worse than I had when I first left my job.

At this point I didn't have many diagnoses, at least not compared to what I have today. I still supposedly had IBS, but I had come to realize that that was wrong. I had undifferentiated connective tissue disease and polycystic ovarian syndrome (PCOS). PCOS is pretty common in Ashkenazi women like me and in certain other ethnic groups, and is not all that uncommon in the population at large. My case was not severe, but not mild either, and I definitely suffered from its effects and from the effects of the hormones that I took to manage it. I was still several years away from discovering just how badly my body was reacting to the hormones I was taking.

I had also been diagnosed as hypothyroid from Hashimoto's disease—an autoimmune disease where antibodies attack the thyroid gland—and I was on medication for that. Unfortunately, it took a long time for me to get that diagnosis and I went without treatment for far too long. The doctors kept testing me and telling me the results were normal. Years later I looked at those test results and found that they were actually on the border of being hypothyroid. When the medical standard for the normal range changed, suddenly they said I was hypothyroid. My results did not change, what changed was what they considered to be the normal range. Given the previously borderline results and my symptoms, not to mention my family history, I should have been put on medication years earlier.

Now I know to always check my own test results. Too often a doctor will simply see that nothing was flagged by the computer and they will not look at each individual number carefully or look at them in combination with each other. I now do this myself. Yet even when I was eventually put on thyroid medications, it was nine years later, after doing my own research, that I discovered it was the wrong medication for me. Little did I know that one day my PCOS symptoms would be alleviated when I stopped taking the birth control hormones and finally got on the right thyroid medication.

Three months out of work stretched into four, then five. I had to return to work at the end of six months unless I filed for long-term disability, and I kept thinking I would go back to work. Finally, though, I had to admit to myself that I would not be going back to work yet and that I had to apply for long-term disability. The nightmare that was the long-term disability application and the following appeal process is a story for another day. The stress of it set back my health to the point that one of my medical practitioners even said there was no point in attempting further treatment until the stress of that process had lessened because my body simply could not handle any more.

It was a horrible process that I would not wish on anyone, and yet, it was necessary for my financial survival, not to mention my physical survival, because being on long-term disability insurance gave me access to my employer's health insurance. I applied for Medicaid but was denied because they claimed that I was not disabled enough. They actually said that I was disabled but not disabled *enough*. Horrifying, isn't it? I went for several months without any health insurance at all and that was terrifying. During this time, I was homebound several days per week. A trip to the grocery store would exhaust me and keep me stuck at home for at least a day. Socializing was often more than I could manage. My life had changed drastically, but I was too ill to see that. Instead, I was busy surviving day to day.

Then one day I was at the library, sitting in a quiet area in the nonfiction section. Randomly, I thought that maybe I should look at a book about IBS—I have no idea why I suddenly had that thought, but thank goodness I did. I walked over to the section on medical issues and a title caught my eye: *Why Do I Still Have Thyroid Symptoms? When My Lab Tests Are Normal* by Datis Kharrazian. I didn't know much about thyroid symptoms at the time; I was as uneducated about them as most people who just listen to their doctors and unquestioningly follow their advice. I haven't made that mistake since that day. Now I do my own research.

That book led me to other books. The reading was torturous. I was so fatigued that I would fall asleep after two pages and then wake up having forgotten what I had read. The brain fog was horrible and I had trouble focusing. My mind would wander. I had trouble understanding the concepts. I was a highly intelligent, highly educated person who could barely manage to read a single chapter. I slogged through that first book and found that subsequent books got easier as I slowly understood the concepts and the biology. I learned that I was not taking the correct medication and that I was not taking necessary supplements. I learned that I wasn't seeing the right kind of doctor. I researched. I coughed up the money for a naturopath who I still see and who changed my life in amazing ways. I got new doctors, though that took longer because the doctor I most wanted to see was not yet covered by my health insurance. When that office began to take my insurance, I quickly made an appointment with that doctor, who I still see. In my few good hours each week, I continued to do my research while dealing with the long-term disability appeal and Social Security filings and all sorts of other government benefits issues that sucked up my time, energy, and brain power. Slowly but surely, I did the work.

My health improved incrementally, and as it did, I was able to do more research. It was during that initial round of research that I realized I needed to stop eating gluten. The rates of gluten intolerance and celiac disease are very high amongst those with Hashimoto's disease. I asked my doctor to test me for celiac disease and she refused, stating that I was just buying into the current fad. She ignored the gastrointestinal symptoms that I had been having for seventeen years. She did give me a referral to a nutritionist and with that nutritionist's help, I went gluten free. It was amazing how quickly I noticed results. Okay, it was actually really slow; it took several months for any change at all. But compared to seventeen years, it felt fast. I was still having a lot of problems but I knew I was on the right track. Sadly, I will never be sure if I have celiac disease because the only way to test it is to eat gluten every day for six to eight weeks, and even kissing someone who ate or drank gluten-containing foods makes me so incredibly ill that I won't consider the test.

I was fortunate to be able to see a world-renowned celiac specialist several years after going gluten free. He looked at my symptoms and at how sensitive I am to gluten, like how I was recently very sick because somebody picked up some grapes, put them down and then I ate those grapes, not knowing they had been touched after they were washed. It was several days of pure hell, followed by two more weeks before I could eat normally. Given my level of sensitivity, and all of my other autoimmune diseases, this specialist told me to consider myself celiac. He agreed it was ridiculous to even attempt to test someone like me because I would be so ill. I wish I knew for sure, but it doesn't change the fact that I have to avoid the slightest trace of gluten contamination. This stresses me out. I am grateful for my rheumatologist who suggested I go gluten free, while feeling bitter that she was unable to test me because her hospital did not allow her to run tests outside of her specialty. What kind of "health" care is that? I am grateful for my own research and for finally going gluten free on my own, though bitter that my primary care physician did not run the necessary tests when I asked her to. The celiac specialist did run the tests, but they came back negative because at that point I had been strictly gluten free for more than a year.

While changing my diet, doing my own research, and dealing with bureaucratic paperwork, I saw more doctors, received more diagnoses, and began more treatments. I was diagnosed with and treated for central sleep apnea, and finally stopped waking up in the morning feeling more exhausted than when I had gone

228

to bed the night before. I found more foods I had to avoid, like corn, broccoli, kale, and peanuts, and others I had to limit, like tomatoes and dairy. These changes help, but they're not enough. I am still too sick to work, too sick to travel, too sick to socialize the way my peers do. This week I saw a new specialist and had twenty vials of blood drawn, all in the hope of finding a new diagnosis, something that could be treated so that I will feel better. Because that's what this is all about: the quest to feel as good as I possibly can.

I will never be healthy. It has taken me a long time to accept that. Some days I acknowledge that reality with understanding and grace. Other days I whine, cry, and lament: Why me? But I know that no matter how I feel about it, it's my reality. I can not change the fact that I will never be healthy, but I can continue to work toward feeling less sick. In small ways, it's working.

This book has taken me six years to publish. Some of that delay was due to life getting in the way or procrastination, but most of it was health-related. I have had to work on this book in increments of just one to two hours, because I can't manage more than that in a day. I have tried to work part-time jobs from home more than once, and each time I got sicker. On the other hand, my gastrointestinal issues, which sometimes had me curled in a ball on the bathroom floor, seriously wondering if death might not be so bad, have improved drastically. I haven't had a migraine in several years. My joint pain is bad, but more days than not it's what I consider to be manageable. My fatigue is still bad, but less bad than it had been. I celebrate every improvement, no matter how small.

Improving my health is an ongoing process that I will struggle with for the rest of my life. It is not easy. Some days I question if I can do it, but I know that for me there is no choice. This is hard shit, and I won't lie about that. But I push through, and I am grateful for the improvements that I have found, even while I struggle constantly.

I know that I have many advantages. I struggle to deal with bureaucratic red tape and wonder how others manage it. I used to deal with this kind of thing for a living, so I have more skills to handle it than most. I am white and well-educated. I speak with good grammar and know how to work within the system. Yet this system is rigged against us. I could write an entire book telling you the many ways that our social safety nets don't catch us here in the United States (and I hear similar stories from patients in other countries, as well). We fall through those big holes that are too rarely acknowledged.

My life changed because I took control of my own medical health. I read my own records, I get every test result and analyze it myself. I put every test result into a spreadsheet and I filter on the test so that I can see the results over time. I Google them. I find new doctors the minute I think that a doctor is not serving my best interests. This is not easy. Not everybody can do it. One day I won't be able to do it and that terrifies me. Right now, I have a list on my computer of things I want to try in an effort to improve my health: supplements, prescriptions, tests, and new types of doctors. Some of these were suggested by doctors, some through my own research, and some by other patients I speak with online. It's important to be careful when speaking with other patients, but I filter the information and then do my own research.

Chronic illness is exhausting because, after all, it is chronic. There is no getting away from it. I want to take a vacation from my health, to get away from it all for a few days, but that's not possible; in fact, travel makes things even more difficult, and I feel worse for many days after even a short trip. And there is no getting away from the discrimination, the stereotypes, or the lack of accessible spaces. I can't get rid of my chronic illnesses, but I am doing the best I can to deal with them and to make it as bearable as possible. After all, what are the alternatives?

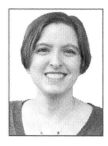

Julie Morgenlender is a friend, daughter, aunt, crocheter, reader, creator of this anthology, and so much more, despite being unable to work full time. She enjoys walking in the sunshine, petting dogs, and spending time with awesome people. She volunteers for her chronic pain support group and is on the board of directors of the Bisexual Resource Center.

Acknowledgements

ONCE I GOT STARTED, this book took six years to publish—and it was in my mind for many years before I began. It was a long process, but worth the effort, and there have been so many people along the way who have helped me, each in their own wonderful way.

My parents, Barbara and David Morgenlender, have been supportive from the start, as they have been with most of my projects throughout my life and I am so appreciative of that. Thank you, Mom and Dad.

Some friends feel like family. Alexandra Wright, Hanna Neier, Marisha Marks, and Miriam Leigh, thank you for all of your support—and the occasional kick in the butt.

To the incredible authors who have shared their lives with us, your writing makes this book everything I had hoped and more. By writing your truths, you are supporting countless others who have so often wondered, "Am I the only one?" Thank you for showing them that they are not alone.

Thank you also to the dozens of writers who submitted stories that were not included within these pages. I appreciate the work you put into your writing, and I only wish I could have included more.

I learned a lot from those who have self-published before me. Robyn Ochs provided knowledge about her own experiences creating anthologies. Robbie Samuels and Doug Hull gave me tips for self-publishing a book. Erik Heels supplied legal advice. Your contributions helped me to create this anthology, and I thank you for your assistance.

One day, as I chatted with a friend of a friend, I mentioned this project. On the spot, she gave me a huge amount of spectacular advice. I hadn't known she was an expert on self-publishing, and I happily hired her for some additional coaching. Thank you so much to Tanya Gold, whose invaluable expertise made a huge impact on this book and on my ability to finish it.

Special thanks to the professional editors who volunteered their time. Nicole Jean Turner spent well over one hundred hours selflessly copyediting this book, making the words sing. Thank you to Nicole for your incredible work, and to Ahna Phillips who provided additional crucial copyediting to make these stories flow. Marie Haaland stepped up when I needed additional help. Her countless time and effort copyediting this book are what pulled it together in the end, giving it a cohesive feel while maintaining each author's voice. Thank you, Marie, for sharing your talents.

Kate Estrop did a fantastic job formatting this book for both print and ebook formats. Bob Thibeault designed a gorgeous cover. Many thanks to each of you for your amazing work.

Thank you to the excellent proofreaders who caught the final typos in this book.

Choosing which stories to include in this book was challenging, and I struggled to narrow down the excellent pieces that were submitted. Thank you to Tanya Saunders for reading all of the submissions, giving your input, and letting me bounce ideas off of you.

For many years, I told myself that I would start this anthology project as soon as I felt well enough. For a long time, I was on a scary health decline. Then, slowly, through my own research and the help of some excellent medical professionals, I began to improve, until finally I was able to create this book. It was still slow going, and sometimes I didn't work on it for months at a time, but I did it. Thank you so much to Angela Weiss, Dr. Gwendolyn Kane-Wanger, Nicole LaRocque, Dr. Guy Pugh, Dr.

June Shibley, and Dr. Robert Thomas. You don't know how much you changed my life. I will be forever grateful for what you did, when so many others had given up.

Creating a project like this can be lonely and overwhelming. A big thank you to Pam McKenna and Jane Lesley for your constant support. You don't know how much you helped me.

Once upon a time I looked for support groups, before finally giving up. I didn't have a mainstream diagnosis, so none of the groups were for me. Then one day, a friend read about a support group for people with chronic pain, and that group changed my life. Thank you to Cindy Steinberg for creating a warm, friendly, and safe environment for me and for so many others. Thank you also to all of the members of that group.

Finally, a huge thank you to the many people out there with chronic illness. Thank you for being there, for reading this book, and for sharing this book with others so that more people will understand what it is like to live with chronic illness.

Bonus: How to Complete a Big Project While Living with Chronic Illness

Do you have a big project that you're having trouble completing, or even starting? Sometimes big projects feel impossible when we're dealing with symptoms, treatments, medical appointments, and more. In this bonus, I break down how I created this book while dealing with my own multiple chronic illnesses. You will learn my initial approach, what worked, what didn't, and how I overcame obstacles, including how I handled the times I felt like giving up.

When you sign up for the bonus, you will also receive the latest on new versions of this book (including the audiobook and video interviews with the authors), sale books, and any new books that are published. (Note: I won't share your email address and you can unsubscribe at any time.)

Get your free copy today at chronicillnesstruths.com/bonus.

Not All Disabilities
Look the Same

I GET TIRED OF people making assumptions about my abilities based on how I look or act at any given moment. One day I shared a meme about invisible disabilities online, and someone asked me if I had a bumper sticker of the image. I explained that it wasn't my design—then I thought, why not make one myself?

I came up with the concept, then hired a graphic designer, Kate Estrop, to do the illustration. That is how this design[9] came to exist on bumper stickers, shirts, water bottles, tote backs, jewelry, and more. I love this design and wear it and carry it often. I get a lot of compliments from people who understand and appreciate why it is so necessary to proclaim that not all disabilities look the same! Get yours at the link below today. If you don't see this design on the product you want, email julie@chronicillnesstruths.com and I will attempt to make it for you.

zazzle.com/chronicillnesstruths

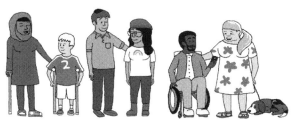

Not all disabilities look the same
chronicillnesstruths.com

---

9 The design is printed in color on all products.

Did You Like This Book?

PLEASE TAKE A MOMENT to visit amazon.com and leave a review. More 5-star reviews will lead to more people reading this book and understanding life with chronic illness.

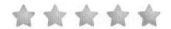

About the Editor

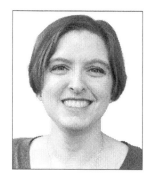

ASIDE FROM MEDICAL APPOINTMENTS for the then-undiagnosed pain she experienced, Julie Morgenlender had a fairly typical 1980s Boston-area childhood of scraped knees and lanyard keychains. Later, she got her bachelor's degree from the University of Massachusetts, Amherst and her master's degree in linguistics from The University of California, Los Angeles—she clearly liked universities with long names. Julie spent her short career in nonprofit organizations before becoming too ill for office work. She then attempted self-employment before realizing she was too ill for that as well.

Julie does not remember when or how she first thought of compiling this anthology, but once the idea took hold, she could not let it go. After nearly a lifetime of feeling alone and misunderstood, she felt it was vitally important to share the hard truths about life with chronic illnesses. It took her six years to create and publish this book, and she is glad she did it.

Julie lives in the Boston area and can be found walking up to strangers and asking to pet their dogs, crocheting on the subway, and sitting in medical practitioners' waiting rooms. She can also be found at the following links:

chronicillnesstruths.com

julie@chronicillnesstruths.com

chronicillnesstruths.com/contact

Glossary

WOULD YOU LIKE TO LEARN what the various terms in this book mean? For definitions and links to useful resources, check out the glossary at chronicillnesstruths.com/glossary.

Index

congenital heart defect, 67

congenital, 55, 204

connective tissue disorder, 45, 75, 77, 78, 221, 222, 225

constipation, 163

coping, 21, 40, 64, 91, 110, 133, 138, 142, 157, 161, 175, 179, 193, 218

Crohn's disease, 60, 153, 159, 211, 212, 217, 218

crutches. *See* mobility aid

cyberchondria, 123

degenerative disc disease, 217

dehydration, 93, 211

depression, 4, 26, 58, 69, 86, 88, 101, 103, 108, 137-139, 217. *See also* five stages of grief cycle. *See also* suicidal ideation

postpartum, 27-30

deterioration, 36, 57, 139

diagnosis, 73, 76, 106, 161, 163, 167, 177, 188-189, 217

delayed, 1, 77, 86, 88, 93-94, 123-124, 141, 153, 219, 222

misdiagnosed, 77-78, 86-87, 217, 219-221, 225

receiving, 8, 22, 26, 40, 45, 80-81, 93-94, 96, 108, 118, 153, 161, 163, 188, 204, 213, 222, 225, 228

undiagnosed, 1, 60-61, 77-80, 142, 188, 217, 219, 225, 239

diet, 22, 36, 40, 47, 62, 142-145, 214, 224, 228-229

disability, 13, 45, 46, 52, 57, 61, 66, 68, 93-94, 97-99, 119-121, 132-135, 143, 180, 185, 188, 208-210, 224-226

disability benefits, 140, 183-187, 207, 226-227, 230. *See also* Social

Security Disability Insurance (SSDI)

disability justice theory, 97, 100

disability pride, 97, 100

disembarkment syndrome, 217

dissociation, 63, 145

dizziness, 93, 190

doctors. *See* medical professionals

dysautonomia, 83, 94, 95. *See also* postural orthostatic tachycardia syndrome (POTS)

dyslexia, 141

Ehlers-Danlos syndrome, 25, 118, 172

Eli Clare, 97

emotions, 29, 31, 62-64, 175, 177

acceptance, 19, 25, 45, 61, 66, 91, 113, 125, 137, 150, 157, 171, 220, 229. *See also* five stages of grief cycle

anger, 8, 14, 63-64, 71, 91, 94, 123, 137-139, 175, 206, 218. *See also* five stages of grief cycle

anxiety. *See* anxiety

avoidance, 62-63

compassion, 42, 104, 106, 110, 112, 149-150, 157, 200, 216

confusion, 2, 48, 49, 61, 78, 109, 122, 175

defeat, 69, 123, 157

denial, 46-47, 124, 137, 139, 157, 185. *See also* five stages of grief cycle

depression. *See* depression

determination, 11. *See also* willpower

disappointment, 12, 62, 111

discouragement, 94, 155

emotions, cont.

    doubt, 1, 78-79, 129, 150, 154, 156, 171, 181, 188

    embarrassment, 12, 90, 160, 163, 205

    failure, 69, 156-157, 167, 206

    fear, 10, 36, 42, 57, 58, 67, 79, 99, 103, 110, 123, 142, 150, 165, 188, 189, 206, 220

    frustration, 1, 29, 58, 64, 77-79, 108, 136, 175, 192, 204, 223

    gratitude, 25, 37-38, 45-46, 48, 64, 87, 116, 139, 145, 147, 150, 164, 192, 222-224, 226, 228-229, 232-234

    grief, 64, 101, 136-139, 170, 222-223. *See also* five stages of grief cycle

    guilt, 10, 38, 47, 158, 199

    happiness, 1, 7, 13, 33, 35, 38-39, 61, 86, 119, 127, 139, 145, 147, 148-149, 161-162, 172, 182, 193, 199, 204

    hope, 3, 7, 9, 15, 24, 29-30, 94, 97, 99, 103-104, 110, 112, 145-146, 171-172, 189, 193, 195, 211-212, 229, 232

    hurt, 22, 25, 35, 64, 78, 91

    isolation, 1-2, 24, 165, 176

    joy, 1, 7, 13, 33, 35, 38-39, 61, 86, 119, 127, 139, 145, 147, 148-149, 161-162, 172, 182, 193, 199, 204

    loneliness, 1, 22, 42, 128, 234

    loss, 47, 101-102, 136-140, 170, 185-186, 222

    love, 7, 9-10, 12, 29-30, 43, 65, 68, 70, 97-99, 118, 127, 137, 157-158, 160, 192-193, 203, 208

emotions, cont.

    panic. *See* anxiety; panic attacks

    positivity, 20, 71, 94-95, 145, 150, 154-155, 157, 160, 169-170

    pride, 97, 133-134, 139, 148, 202, 205-206

    regret, 169

    relief, 62, 112, 188

    resentment, 127, 145

    sadness, 1, 35, 42, 48, 50, 61, 64, 86, 94, 120, 133, 160, 170-171, 175-176, 189, 213-214, 219, 228. *See also* five stages of grief cycle

    shame, 58, 97, 99, 105, 150

    strength, 24, 30, 64-65, 81, 94, 103, 112, 124-125, 128, 157-158, 162, 168, 171, 192, 206, 215

    stress, 17-19, 24, 56-59, 110, 123-124, 148, 222, 226, 228

    worry, 10, 18, 21, 26, 36, 46, 66, 80, 94, 108, 111, 122, 134, 169-170, 217, 221

    worthiness, 71, 87, 98, 154, 157-158, 191

employment, 29, 41, 57-58, 98, 115, 123, 138-139, 183, 194, 208, 219, 220, 222-226, 229, 239

endometriosis, 50, 163

eugenics, 96

exercise, 47, 52, 104-105, 148, 150, 154, 213. *See also* treatments: physical therapy; treatments: physiotherapy

fainting, 68, 118

fatigue, 34, 36, 38-39, 45, 47, 86, 94, 120, 126, 141-142, 144, 163, 190, fatigue, cont., 192, 220, 223-224, 227, 229. *See also* myalgic encephalomyelitis/chronic fatigue syndrome (ME/CFS)

fibromyalgia, 16-17, 26, 40, 79, 127-128, 162, 178, 193, 203, 205, 211-212

finances, 3, 38, 57, 76, 115, 134, 184, 186, 226. *See also* medical bills; money

five stages of grief cycle, 136, 222

fusion. *See* surgery

gallstones, 217

gastroesophageal reflux disease, 95

gastroparesis, 212

generalized anxiety disorder, 16, 108, 122-125. *See also* anxiety

glandular fever, 119, 133-134

glycogen storage disease type XI, 95

government benefits. *See* disability benefits

Hashimoto's disease, 225, 227

headache, 163

hiatal hernia, 141

Hidradenitis suppurativa, 163

hospitals, 26-29, 33, 53, 61-62, 66-72, 73, 83-84, 88, 93, 98, 104 119, 159, 164, 175-176, 212, 228

hypermobility, 80

hyperventilating, 109

hypervigilance, 63

hypothyroid, 225-226

infertility, 37, 49-50

inflammatory bowel disease, 159

insomnia, 101, 108

insurance, 29, 38, 48, 70, 76, 78, 164, 220, 226-227. *See also* Social Security Disability Insurance (SSDI)

interstitial cystitis, 163

invalidation. *See* validation

invisible disability, 58, 180, 182. *See also* invisible illness

invisible illness, 38, 40-41, 43, 46-47, 58, 67, 122, 160-161, 180, 182, 194, 211-212, 217, 236. *See also* invisible disability

irritable bowel syndrome, 163, 220-221, 225-226

job. *See* employment

joint dislocation, 120, 166

joint hypermobility syndrome, 193

keratoconus, 56, 59

LGBTQIA+, 2, 16, 20, 39, 51, 76, 82, 97-98, 231

lichen sclerosus, 8-10

light sensitivity, 56-57, 194

liver dysfunction, 141

lupus, 45, 86, 126, 141-144, 146, 221

malaria, 217

malnutrition, 211

Medicaid, 226

medical bills, 164, 206

medical professionals, 8-10, 21, 24, 26-29, 33, 37, 38, 40, 42, 49-51, 60, 62 66-72, 73, 76, 77-80, 83-84, 86-89, 93-94, 96-98, 103-106, 117, 118, 127, 133, 146, 147, 153-156, 158, 161, 163-165, 167-168, 170, 175-176, 181, 184, 188-189, 195, 203, 217-218, 219-222, 225-228, 230

mental health, 21, 28-29, 37, 86-88, 90, 103-104, 108, 110-111, 112, 123-125, 139, 204, 223

medical tests, 37, 40, 42, 44, 45, 60, 77-78, 84, 88, 93-94, 96, 119, 138, 154, 211, 221-222, 225, 227-228, 230

Made in the USA
Columbia, SC
05 June 2025

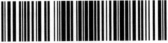